The FEAR Bucket List

From Victim to Power Woman

Dr. Kamilla Holst, D.C.

"This is a fun, interesting book by one courageous woman! It combines adventure travel, spirituality, and a personal journey with originality and passion. It will inspire many to overcome their own fears."
Cloe Madanes – Bestselling author and President, Robbins-Madanes Training

"This is a fun, interesting book by one courageous woman! It combines adventure travel, spirituality, and a personal journey with originality and passion. It will inspire many to overcome their own fears."

Cloé Madanes – President, Robbins-Madanes Training, bestselling author

"This is a great book! It's full of whit and wisdom. If you've ever wondered how you will conquer what you are afraid of, this is the book to read. Kamilla has done it all, and come through feeling her fear, and doing it anyway! Bravo, for a great story, but KUDOS for conquering her fears. You'll be afraid right along with her—and wonder how she did it! You'll read it and decide you can too!"

Maureen St. Germain –Author, mystic, and world thought leader

"Kamilla Holst was struggling with fear, and she won the battle. The author of this book was willing to take action and get her hands dirty in the pursuit to set herself free. By sharing her story, she demonstrates how you can change your life by empowering yourself. All you need in order to be "released" from your own mental prison is to decide for yourself that you will not let your fear dictate your future."

Sofia Manning – Coach and bestselling author

"The deeply empowering and wonderfully uplifting *The Fear Bucket List* by Kamilla Holst opens the doorways to overcoming and conquering your fears as you journey with her around the world! I really loved the personal insight of mastering the emotional self as Kamilla takes you deep into the jungles of the human spirit and out through the enlightened passageways in the Egyptian deserts. This powerful account builds upon your character with every chapter and gently guides the reader towards what it means to embrace the strength and power within us all."

Sufian Chaudhary – Creator and author of *World of Archangels*

"A deeply personal, courageous, and honest insight into the intentional and life-long journey that is overcoming trauma and fear. In a world often filled with stigma and prejudice around survivors of abuse, this book offers a message of hope and self-empowerment to those who no longer want to be defined by the trauma of their past."

Melissa Petros – Executive Director Hagar International (Hong Kong)

The
FEAR
Bucket List

From Victim to Power Woman

Dr. Kamilla Holst, D.C.

DrHolst@TheFearBucketList.com

www.TheFearBucketList.com

www.kamillaholst.com

Published by Kamilla Holst Ltd.

Copyright © 2017 by Dr. Kamilla Holst

The stories in this book have been reprinted with permission from the individuals involved. In some cases, names and identifying details have been changed to preserve confidentiality.

All rights reserved. No parts of this book may be reproduced by any mechanical, photographic, or electronic process, or in the form of a phonographic, or electronic recording; nor may it be stored in a retrieval system, transmitted, or otherwise be copied for public or private use – other than for "fair use" as brief quotations embodied in articles and reviews without prior written permission of the publisher.

The author of this book does not dispense medical advice or prescribe the use of any technique as a form of treatment for physical or medical problems without the advice of a physician, either directly or indirectly. The intent of the author is only to offer information of a general nature to help you in your quest for emotional and spiritual well-being. In the event you use any of the information in this book yourself, which is your constitutional right, the author and the publisher assume no responsibility for your actions.

Limit of liability: While the publisher and author have used their best efforts in preparing this book, they make no representations or warranties with respect to the accuracy or completeness of the contents of this book and specifically disclaim any implied warranties of merchantability or fitness for a particular purpose. No warranty may be created or extended by sales representatives or written sales materials. The advice and strategies contained herein may not be suitable for your situation. You should consult with a professional where appropriate. Neither the publisher nor author shall be liable for any loss of profit or any other commercial damages, including but not limited to special, incidental, consequential, or other damages.

For print or media interviews with Kamilla please contact DrHolst@TheFearBucketList.com

ISBN-13: 978-1522881186

ISBN-10: 1522881182

Cover design: Ken Leeder

This book is dedicated to the millions of victims out there who have suffered from fear and abuse of any kind.

I have decided to donate 100% of the book's proceeds to the non-profit organization Hagar International that specializes in restoring and empowering women and children in Afghanistan, Cambodia, and Vietnam whose lives have been devastated by extreme human rights abuses—particularly domestic violence, exploitation, and human trafficking.

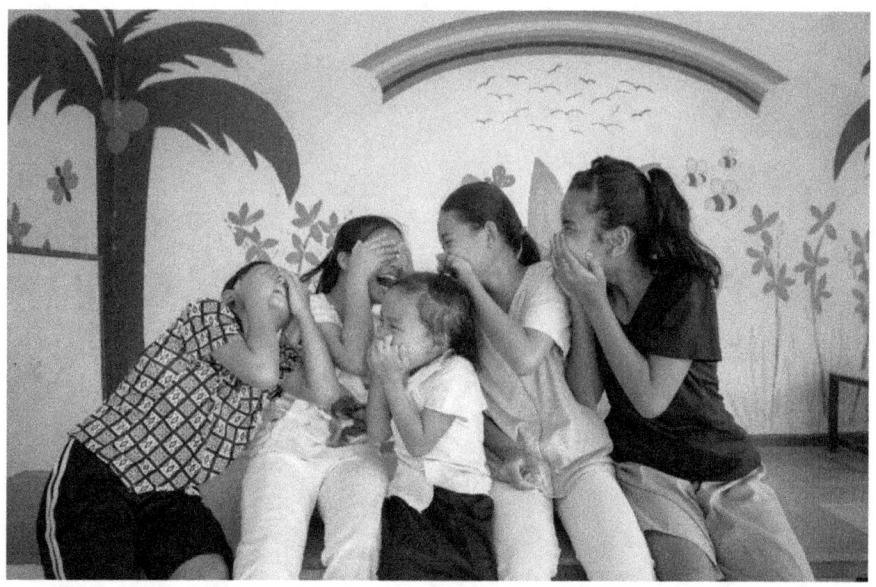

Copyright © 2017 Hagar International

CONTENTS

Introduction 1

PART I – Fear 7

Chapter 1: What Is Fear? 9
    Fear, according to the scientists 9
    How do you turn your fear into power? 12
    Fear, according to the indigenous people 18
    Fear, according to a tai chi master 19

Chapter 2: Our Own Worst Enemy 21
    Body/mind correlation 26
    Case studies 28

Chapter 3: How Fear Can Affect Our Health 33

PART II – From the Beginning 39

Chapter 4: Learning How to Swim the Frogman Way 41

Chapter 5: When Everything Changed – The Effects of Sexual Abuse 45

Chapter 6: Date with Destiny 59

PART III – In the Footsteps of the Initiates 67

Chapter 7: Egypt 69
    Temple of Hathor 71
    Kom Ombo 76

Chapter 8: Mexico 81
    Chakras 82
    Crystal skull ceremony 91

Chapter 9: Spirituality 101 95

Chapter 10: Meditation 103

Part IV – The Fear Bucket List **113**

Chapter 11: Fear of White Sharks 115

Chapter 12: Fear of Small Spaces (Cave Diving) 119

Chapter 13: Fear of Heights 125

Chapter 14: Fear of Crashing 131

Chapter 15: Fear of Being Alone 135

Chapter 16: Fear of Not Being Good Enough 139

Chapter 17: Fear of Public Speaking 143

Bonus: Advice from a Danish Singer 147

Conclusion 153

This Is Not the End. It Is the Beginning! 155

References 165

Acknowledgments 167

About Hagar International 169

About Dr. Kamilla Holst 171

Introduction

Globally, it is estimated that twenty percent of women and five to ten percent of men alive today were sexually abused as children.[1] And that is just an estimate. So many victims keep their abuse a secret, just like I did, and are not part of the statistics.

Common symptoms are shame, self-blame, depression, anxiety, post-traumatic stress disorder, self-esteem issues, sexual dysfunction, chronic pelvic pain, addiction, self-injury, suicidal thoughts, borderline personality disorder, and tendency to re-victimization in adulthood.

No child should ever have to go through anything like this, but, unfortunately, many do around the world every single day.

Do you ever think about how carefree and fearless children are? They don't think about the consequences all the time, they jump right in and experience life. Adults seem to have forgotten this feeling. Why is that? Life happens, traumas

---

[1] *Source: www.arkofhopeforchildren.org*

occur, we make key decisions in situations that affect the rest of our lives.

I believe FEAR is the primary power that stops a person from developing spiritually. It keeps you from becoming awakened to live a happy productive life. Therefore, I have made it one of my life's goals to overcome my fears in order to raise my level of consciousness and self-awareness.

Everyone has fears. It's a natural feeling. But, what separates successful people from ordinary people is that they don't allow their fears to limit or define them. Fear inevitably keeps you in the same position and stops your growth. Recognize your fears and seek ways to overcome them one way or the other.

For me, the journey towards truly living again began with pushing through my fears and pain in order to take back control of my life. Through my personal story, I will demonstrate how facing my fears set me free, and provide encouragement to other women who no longer want to be defined by their past trauma. The book's central message is one of hope and empowerment: **No matter what trauma you have experienced, you have the power to overcome it.**

I know from experience, life is much more interesting when you aren't sabotaging yourself or letting other people bring you down. Life is definitely not boring; it is full of challenges that you need to overcome. No one else can do it for you. *Accept it.* This is part of our life lessons on Earth. If nothing challenged us, we would be bored shitless!

Introduction

I didn't have to write this book, I could have taken my secret to the grave, but I believe in my heart that I was called to help someone else out there, who might have suffered in silence the same way I did for so many years. If I can prevent just one suicide, it will all be worth it. I believe that everything that happened to me happened for a reason and a purpose, and it served to make me the person I am today.

So, how is this book different from all the other self-help books out there?

This book was never supposed to be published. It was a collection of my personal notebooks and research that I wrote down as part of my self-healing journey.

And now it has become my way of giving back and showing anyone in doubt that it *is* possible to go from Victim to Power Woman by facing your fears. 100 % of the book's proceeds will go to a non-profit organization.

I can't wait to share with you all the knowledge and lessons I have learned and collected in the last seven years from all over the world on my quest to overcome my sexual abuse in my own holistic way without any medicine. It is ancient knowledge that will hopefully help you get out of your comfort zone and start living the life you deserve without anything holding you back anymore.

I will be explaining how fear works in the brain (to give you an idea of the physical aspects), I will share techniques on how to conquer your fear, and I will also give you insight into the spiritual realm through my many journeys.

Furthermore, I will be sharing my own personal Fear Bucket List with you and how it changed my life forever.

You have probably heard about or seen the 2007 movie *The Bucket List* with Morgan Freeman and Jack Nicholson. In that movie, they describe a bucket list as a list of things you want to do before you die.

When I saw the movie with these two old men on their death beds, planning to do all the things on their list, I realized why wait. Why not go out and face your fears now? What would the rest of your life be like, if you started facing your fears now instead of when you were old?

Normally, a bucket list also includes all the pleasant things you want to try before you die, but I figured if I wanted to really change my life, I needed to do only the unpleasant and scary things, and that is how The Fear Bucket List came to life.

With this book and by sharing my story and Fear Bucket List with you, I want to send a message that you are not alone; it is never too late to get help. I'm hoping that I can encourage you to break the silence, speak out, and do something to change your life by empowering yourself and step out of the victim role, no matter what happened to you.

So, my wish for you, before you continue with this book, is to make the commitment, to take responsibility for your own life, and do what it takes to change your path. Are you ready for this?

Please affirm with a big vibrant YES!

Introduction

***

Before we go any further, please set your intention for reading this book in order to get the most out of it. You might not have experienced exactly the same as me, but you will still get a lot out of the principles of this book if you set your mind to it.

An intention can be anything from *"I will read this book with an open heart"* to *"I'm taking this time for myself "* or *"I'm ready to change."* Whatever it is for you, make the intention before you read any further.

Close your eyes and take three deep breaths, connect to your heart, feel it beating in your chest, feel gratitude for it beating without you having to tell it to, feel the gratitude in your core that you are still here today, and then state your intention out loud.

Did you do it? Did you make your intention? <u>If not, go back and do it!!!</u>

Now we can continue. ☺

To live the life you want, you need to know <u>what</u> you want! The more positive and specific you can define it, the easier it is for your subconscious mind to notice possibilities in your everyday life.

You don't need to stay a victim; you can change your life today.

There is no right or wrong way to overcome fear or abuse. This is just my own personal way.

Some people might need professional therapy. In fact, I encourage you to seek help if anything has happened to you. I didn't choose that option for myself. I decided on a more holistic way to deal with it on my own. Remember, everyone is different.

It's up to you to choose the road that suits your needs and manifests your own reality.

This is my way ....

I have created **The Fear Bucket List workbook** for you to fill out in your own time.

Download it HERE

www.TheFearBucketList.com

PART I – Fear

Chapter 1:
What Is Fear?

Fear, according to the scientists

According to the scientists, fear is an unconscious biological response that stems from having deeply rooted beliefs that something or someone will cause you to have physical, mental, emotional, spiritual, or financial harm.

Let me give you an example:

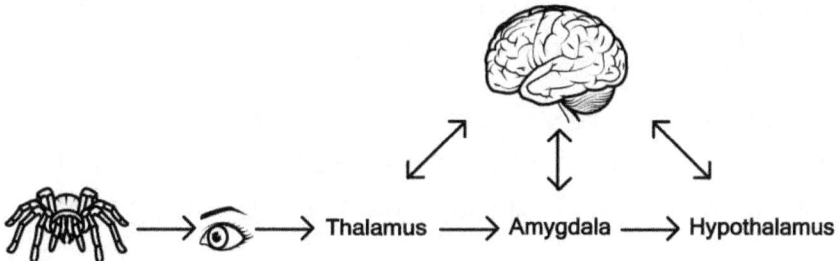

Fear trigger response in the brain

External stimuli or internal thoughts can trigger a response—for example, a human sees a spider.

This information is directed through the eyes to the part of the brain called the *thalamus*. The thalamus is a midline symmetrical structure of two halves, within the vertebrate brain, situated between the cerebral cortex and the midbrain. Some of its functions are the relaying of sensory and motor signals to the cerebral cortex, and the regulation of consciousness, sleep, and alertness. [2]

From there, the information is sent directly to the *prefrontal cortex* and becomes the actual notion of "I'm seeing a spider!" The cortex covers the majority of the human brain and is between 1.5 mm and 5 mm thick. The cortex is split in two halves: a front part and a back part. The back part deals with "Where am I?" meaning it analyzes the sensory information. The front part deals with "What do I do?" It controls the motoric action involved.[3]

The information is also sent to the *amygdala*, and there the emotional reaction is being coordinated. The amygdala has the shape and size of an almond. It coordinates the body's emotional response with our conscious feelings and is primarily active in a threatening situation.[4]

The amygdala speaks with the *hypothalamus* and the body reacts.[5] The hypothalamus plays a central role in the basic brain functions like urges and instincts. It is responsible for

---

[2] ***Thalamus:*** *Dr. Zukovs Testamente*
[3] *Cortex: Netter's Atlas of Anatomy.*
[4] *Amygdala: Wikipedia*
[5] *Hypothalamus: Netter's Atlas of Anatomy.*

Chapter 1: What is Fear?

the overall coordination of the emotional response of the body.

At the same time, the amygdala speaks with the cortex where the feeling of "I'm in danger" and all the potential future consequences lie. You become aware of the fact that you are scared.

The science shows us that this response system has been part of our human brains for as long as we have existed and hasn't developed much since. It developed in a time when there was a good reason to be scared. Lots of dangerous things could happen to us at all times, and we needed to survive. *It is there to protect you. So, it's not really your fault when you feel fearful!*

This response system is part of the basic brain functions—the primitive parts of your brain, so to speak. It is also called the reptilian brain.

What naturally happens when you feel frightened is automatic: the body jumps, you might scream, your heart starts pumping really fast, your mouth becomes dry, your breathing becomes more frequent and shallow, you start sweating, and your stress hormones get activated. Basically, the brain prepares you to ***fight or flight***. The fight or flight response is a physiological reaction that occurs in response to a perceived harmful event, attack, or threat to survival.[6] This means your body is preparing to fight the tiger or run away from it.

---

[6] **Wikipedia**

The Fear Bucket List

What you do from there is the key. Fear will affect your decision making, thinking abilities, solution finding, etc. So, **unless you turn your fear into power**, your response is going to be exactly the same every time.

How do you turn your fear into power?

To answer this question, I interviewed the one person I figured would know the most about fearful situations, my father, Georg H. Petersen (Putte), a legend in the Danish Frogman Corps with survival as his area of expertise. He is an author, and he has received countless medals.

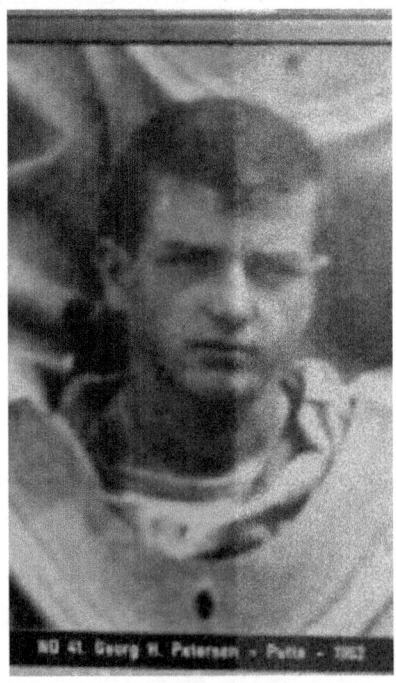

Georg H. Petersen 'Putte' 1962

Chapter 1: What is Fear?

"What do you usually tell your boys about fear?"

Putte: "When I brief the frogmen about fear, I tell them it's okay to be afraid, even for a frogman, but, the minute you feel scared, *the minute fear arrives, you have to acknowledge it and say 'fine'*!

"Maybe you've fallen from a plane with your parachute and landed in enemy territory, or fallen into an ambush, or something like that (it can be many scenarios), but the moment the fear occurs, you have to *ask yourself, 'Can I magically make the fear disappear?'* You probably can't. *'How do I get on from here?'* The fear will not dissolve by itself. So, instead of being paralyzed by it and not doing anything, find out what you CAN do to survive.

"It is so important to be aware of this, especially those men in the Special Forces who will not admit to being scared.

"Being afraid or fearful is a natural human reaction like being hungry or tired. It is a natural thing. Everyone has been afraid. If a person refuses to acknowledge that they are afraid, at some point they will break down. Instead, <u>recognize the fear,</u> <u>work with it,</u> and <u>do something</u> in the present situation! That is the most important lesson."

"Okay, I'm scared shitless. So what!? How do I move on?"

"Have you ever been SO afraid that you couldn't say to yourself 'How do I move on from this'?"

Putte: "I was terrified once. I was standing on the bottom of a lake about sixty-six meters down with a brass helmet on (weighing ninety kilos), and I couldn't breathe.

13

The Fear Bucket List

"I had lost my search line and couldn't get back to the diving platform.

"At this depth, you can only stay for about five minutes, and then you need to ascend to avoid decompression sickness. So, I thought *What am I going to do now?* I told the ship above that I had lost my search line and suggested that my buddy 'Busk' should walk back to the platform, and then from there walk out thirty meters, tie his search line to my dropped one, and then go out sixty meters in total and do a big circle until he bumped into me. And he did! Back then, we couldn't communicate directly, only to the ship above.

"Even though I was terrified, I acknowledged my fear and thought *What do I do now? How do I get myself out of this situation?* I knew it was a really bad situation, but I had to focus on what to do, because every minute staying down there meant half an hour more in the decompression chamber, and the decompression sickness might kill me.

"I ended up being down there only ten minutes too long thanks to my good friend and buddy. But the ascent took over three hours in very cold water and, on top of that, I had nitrogen poisoning,[7] so when I got back to the platform, I managed to tie Busk to it with my line, without even knowing it, until the ship yelled to me saying 'What the hell are you doing to him? He's screaming and shouting!'

"Another dive later on, after we got away from the heavy brass helmets, I ran out of air at forty-one meters. I signaled

---

[7] *Nitrogen Poisoning:* also known as nitrogen narcosis, which causes alteration in consciousness while diving at depth. The narcosis produces a state similar to drunkenness (Wikipedia).

Chapter 1: What is Fear?

my dive buddy to turn on my reserve tank because the water was very cold, and my suit was so insulated that I couldn't reach it myself.

"He didn't understand what I wanted him to do and, in the end, I had to do an emergency ascent and ended up pulling him eight to ten meters with the buddy line before he realized something was wrong and followed me. I remember at some point that I couldn't hold my breath any longer, and I inhaled the cold water. Right away, I told myself that it was a very bad idea and, if I continued doing that, it was over and, instead, I should just continue upwards. I don't know how, but I got up to the surface.

"When I got my breath back, I yelled at my buddy because he didn't help me, but all he could say was 'Oh, I thought you had seen a shark!' Later on, he dropped out of the training.

"There was another incident when the hair on my neck rose. Back in 1991, I was stationed in Croatia where the Serbians had occupied the city I was in. We had been strictly told not to move outside on our own; we had to be two together. But they didn't say anything about running, so I decided to put on my running shoes and go for an early morning run. After about seven kilometers, I noticed that there were shells on the ground. I slowed down and noticed that I was in the middle of no man's land.

"This was when my hair stood up on the back of my neck. I realized I was a human target. I turned around and sprinted as fast as I could. It was a strange feeling, because I was aware that something was not quite right … there were no people … no birds singing …

"It was the same feeling I've gotten a few times when bullets have been fired at me. The feeling of a bullet just flying over your head … it's really something that makes your hair stand up!

"Once, I was on a half island being chased by soldiers. The island became more and more narrow, and there was no return. Moving forward seemed to be the only option. So, instead of letting my fear take over and just run, I decided to stop and camouflage myself in a rose bush.

"I walked backwards into the bush and hid, motionless, about twenty centimeters in. The first German Shepard dog came along and was standing right in front of me eyeballing me. I stayed completely still, but the dog kept barking. Five minutes later, a soldier came and pulled the dog away saying 'You stupid dog; no one's in there!' That was a close call! Looking at that dog barking at me with froth around its mouth and teeth showing was not a pleasant sight.

"Another time, I was skydiving with the commando troops. I had jumped out and my parachute released but, while I was hanging there, I saw one of the trooper students head straight towards me! I had to twist and turn, but he continued to steer right at me, so I had to yell at him to turn away, because if he entered the airspace right above me, he would take away my air and my parachute would collapse. I really couldn't have that!

Chapter 1: What is Fear?

"My subconscious was aware in advance that if I didn't get away from him in time, it would end badly, so I yelled at him to steer the opposite to me and, in the end, he got it. *Sometimes you need to try different solutions* until it works, even when you're afraid.

"Fear paralyzes so many people and that it is almost the worst thing that can happen. You can't use that reaction for anything or you will risk dying!

"*Acknowledging your fear is the key*; it will not just go away by itself, and you have to learn how to deal with it when it occurs."

"*What separates the people who react and the people who get paralyzed by fear?*"

Putte: "If they don't know it's natural to feel afraid when they face the situation the first time, most people will become paralyzed. But, if you know it's a natural reaction and accept this, your chances of getting terrified and freezing are less likely.

"If you feel hunger, you don't get paralyzed right? You find some food to eat. So, why get paralyzed when you feel fear? This emotion is just as natural as feeling hungry.

"You might not do the right thing all the time, but at least you are doing SOMETHING! And you will likely get out of that situation. You will be able to think more clearly and be more aware."

The Fear Bucket List

"What happens inside of you when you have experienced all of these close calls and gotten out on the other side? What does that do to you?"

Putte: "I never really thought about that! I think I feel happy that I made it and that I gained some useful experience, so the next time it's much easier to get out of a similar situation. It's a development from where you were to where you are now, a new level of consciousness."

Fear, according to the indigenous people

To get a different perspective about the definition of fear, I asked a Mayan Elder during my stay with them back in 2012 **"What is fear?"**

"Fear happens when you are out of alignment with who you really are, when you forget who you really are. The spirit does not experience fear, only the personality does. Therefore, *if you eliminate fear, you become closer to your spirit in this incarnation.*

That is our ultimate purpose, to align ourselves with our spirit. Most of us just forget about our purpose and get trapped in our everyday lives, thinking that this is our reality, when it's really just an illusion or *maya*.[8]

---

[8] *Maya is the term used by the indigenous people of Yucatan and means illusion.*

Chapter 1: What is Fear?

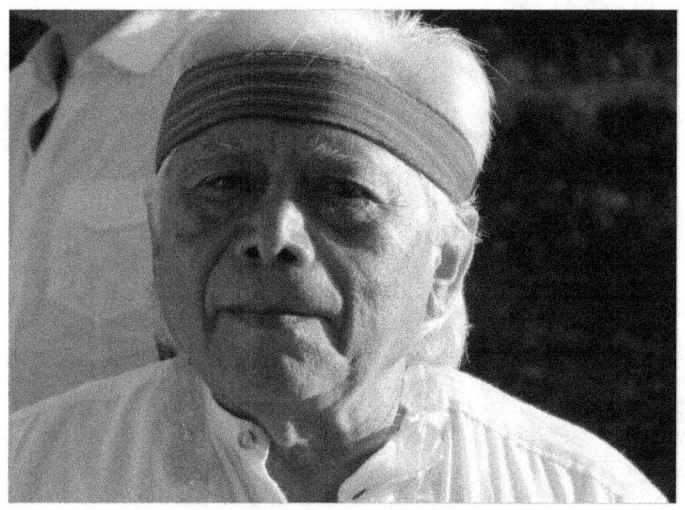

Mayan elder - Hunbatz Men

Fear, according to a tai chi master

I've been studying the ancient art of tai chi for a while, and I asked my teacher how the Taoists define fear.

"Taoism normally doesn't talk about 'fear.' Taoist philosophy talks more about worry and uncertainty in our lives that prevents us from relaxing, and it emphasizes how important it is not to dwell on this emotion. If you know your body well and know what kind of person you are, what is there to fear? If you don't do anything evil to other people, then who is going to come at night and attack you from behind in the darkness? If you're not worried about that, what fear do you have?

The Fear Bucket List

There's a Chinese proverb that says: In your life, if you don't do anything bad to others, then you won't be worried if someone knocks on your door in the middle of the night.

It's a way of living. If you don't do harm to others, you are peaceful in your heart, and there is no need to fear."

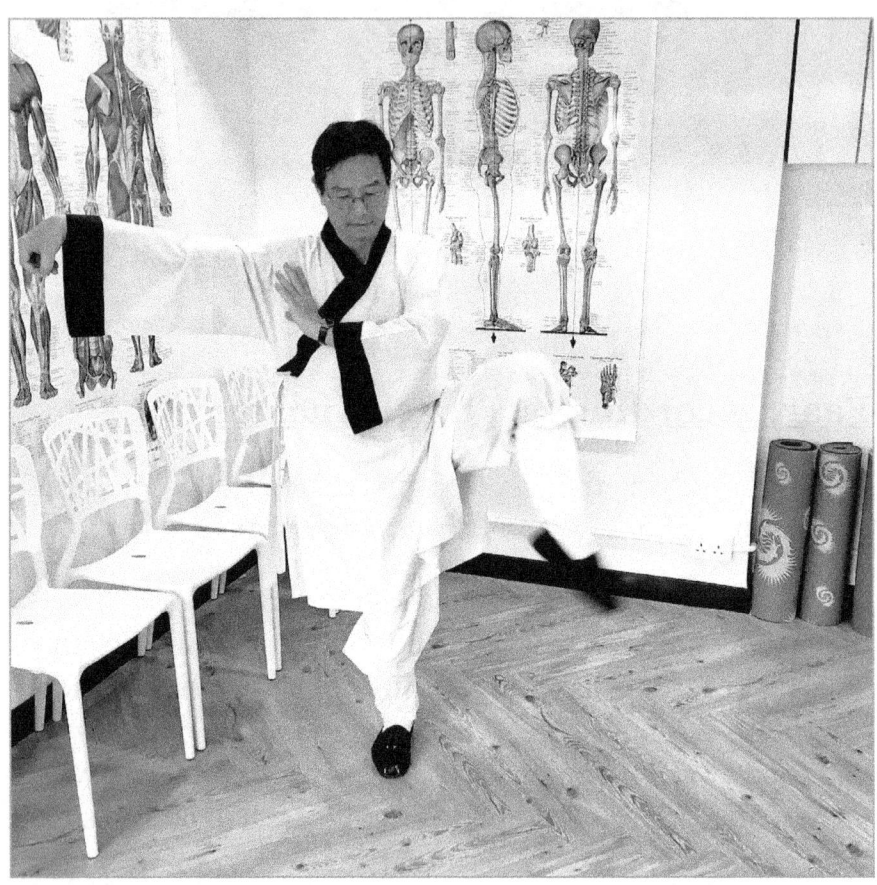

Tai Chi Master – Dr. Benjamin Yip, D.C.

Chapter 2:
Our Own Worst Enemy

In the modern world, you are no longer being chased by wild animals (hopefully), which means your normal day-to-day life is not filled with the same kind of danger as earlier in your evolution. But the part that controls fear in your brain is still the same. There is too little to be scared of, so what you experience now, more than ever, is a pattern of an endless *excess of fear* and worrying about what other people think about you, if you're good enough, and other emotions that don't serve you.

You can be your own best friend or your own worst enemy.

There are so many levels of fear, anxiety being one level of fear. Some people are so afraid that they don't get to enjoy life, because fear is holding them back. They end up wasting a lifetime just to feel safe.

Scientists have shown that we are more inclined to *avoid our fears* than pursue our happiness. This causes people to stay where they are and not expand their level of consciousness. They stay in their comfort zone. They worry about things that haven't happened yet and limit themselves and the people around them. You see, fear is contagious!

The Fear Bucket List

Does this sound familiar? I'll bet you know someone in your life that lives like this, someone who never takes any chances or suffers from regular anxiety.

When we let fear take over, we forget who we really are. When it comes down to it, all we are is love and, when we remember this, there is no reason for fear anymore.

Fear does not exist in the Love Dimension, the fifth dimension that we are slowly entering here on Earth. It is something we create in the third dimension, and it is also called the Dimension of Polarity, where many people are at this moment. Polarity can be described as evil versus good, white versus black, right versus wrong. This is old energy, and we need to move away from this mindset.

Do many people walk around with fear? The answer is YES!

Many of my clients have different kinds of fears; some are more affected than others are, because we are all different and react to trauma in various ways.

Fear is part of being a human. So, why even spend time writing about fear—because fear is ingrained in us, and it is time for you to have the courage to burn through your fears and set your mind and body free.

Have you ever noticed how the media thrives on telling us stories that make us worry? It's not possible to see a news report without some sort of crisis or disease somewhere in the world.

What concerns me is the way a message is delivered nowadays. To give you an example: in the past, you would

Chapter 2: Our Own Worst Enemy

be advised to eat a varied diet with fibers in order to "be healthy" now the same message will end with "to avoid colon cancer!" The media have a tendency to add a little fear wherever they can.

Every day the news brings us stories about crumbling finances, deadly diseases, terror, and people dying. The fear is pushed in everywhere, because it works. It keeps people watching and, at the same time, it keeps people suffering.

For me, FEAR has always been a part of my life. As far back as I can remember, I was guilty of letting it control my life, until I *found a method to empower myself*: facing the fears on my Fear Bucket List combined with meditation.

Research shows that the number one biggest fear is **_not being good enough_** *(a fear of failure).*[9] Humans want to be good enough and ultimately good enough to be loved and fit in.

I was guilty of thinking that I wasn't old enough to publish a book. I thought no one would take me seriously. So, I waited until I was in my thirties to publish my first book, which is so ridiculous and irrational, and the kind of thinking that can hold you back from doing good in this world. Low self-esteem and fear of what other people might think can hold you back for a lifetime.

We've all been there. "Once I've studied more, I will teach others." "Once I've got enough money, I'll travel or start my

---

[9] *Robbins, Anthony. Unlimited Power. 2008*

own business." "Once I feel comfortable, I will let him in and tell him how I feel." And the list goes on.

What do you think happens if you walk around with this feeling inside of you (or any other fear for that matter) for a long period of time? Nothing good I can tell you.

Every day I see how *the mind is one of our most powerful tools of healing*. But if our minds are cluttered with fears, it doesn't work properly.

The powerful engine that creates healing is your subconscious mind.

You are whole, perfect, and complete, a part of the universal order. You can create your own pain relief. Your words create your world, as *your thinking is your reality*.

If you say things are bad then they are bad. Conversely, if you are present with the good things in your life, and live inside of those things, then life appears completely different. You create a powerful context, and the universe aligns. You have a choice in the matter of how your life will go and the quality of life you want to have.

You have the power within you.

We all have something we fear—not being loved, being abandoned, heights, spiders, snakes, public speaking, fear of success, fear of failure, fear of disappointing yourself, etc.

Bodies react to the thoughts you make. Our psychological and emotional state affects the endocrine system. For example, the emotion of fear is connected to *adrenalin*.

Chapter 2: Our Own Worst Enemy

If no feeling of fear exists, there is no adrenalin and the same applies in reverse—no adrenalin, no fear! They work in relation to each other. Wherever a thought goes, there's a chemical reaction in the body. So, let's start this powerful way of self-healing by being aware of the underlying stream of thoughts.

Most people have experienced some kind of trauma in their life at some point. When I say trauma, I mean an emotional response to a terrible event, it can be anything from a car accident to rape. This can lead to unhappiness if you don't learn how to deal with it.

Be very aware of your feelings. Are you taking responsibility or creating drama and blaming others? What is your pattern?

One of my favorite teachers, **Eckart Tolle,** says it very well:

"The ego needs to be in conflict with something or someone. That explains why you are looking for peace and joy and love but cannot tolerate them for very long. You say you want happiness but are addicted to your unhappiness."

It is human nature to respond and react in a certain way and it is okay. As long as we become aware of this, it opens up a window to change.

Through the years, I have helped many clients notice where they hold the tension in their body, and how they themselves can move it and become self-reliant. You have everything inside of you right now. You have the power to self-heal.

I help people accept their body as a whole unit, not two separate things consisting of a head and a body.

Body/mind correlation

Body/mind correlation is the teaching of how your negative thought patterns affect your body physically and how you take responsibility to turn it around in order to create balance.

This is so important to understand. If you want to change your life, you need to learn how to <u>master your emotions</u>!

If you have any kind of pain—physically, emotionally, mentally, or spiritually—you are probably experiencing a hold on your energy, and you need to learn to release it.

Instead of going through life with pain ... think about it. What signals is your body sending you? What is causing this sensation in your body?

If you wake up with a pain in your neck, most people say they slept on it wrong but, in fact, it's just a buildup of tension ready to be released, it is a symptom that needs investigation. *Pain is often a signal that you are ready to release.*

Often when you experience a traumatic event, this energy or emotion will affect your body physically later on in one way or another. This is a known fact called 'psychosomatic' pain,[10] which basically means mind-body, and it is based on the notion that how you are feeling is reflected in the state of

---

[10] *The British Journal of Psychiatry Dec. 2005, 188 (1) 91-93*

Chapter 2: Our Own Worst Enemy

your body. Some people will feel it as a stomachache, others as a migraine that keeps coming back, tension in the body, ulcers, heart issues, sexual dysfunction, etc. No matter what the trauma, it's possible to work on it and slowly release it from your body.

Once you start releasing this energy, you will feel better. You can do this in many ways. One way is through meditation and awareness of your body and mind. Another is physical release in the form of healing massage, sound healing or chiropractic treatment balancing the interference in your nervous system by removing any or all subluxations[11] in your body that you have accumulated through the years. Or you can go the more traditional way and use psychotherapy.

1) Consider *you* are an energetic being

2) *Understand* what the pain is telling you

The body is just an illusion created by your consciousness so you can have a materialistic experience that is really fun; you get to eat chocolate, dance, sing, laugh, write books, and experience nature on this beautiful planet. It's such a great gift! So, breathe in life and release all your negative energy.

---

[11] *Subluxation: a slight misalignment of the vertebrae regarded in chiropractic theory as the cause of many health problems.*

Case studies

A young woman came to my clinic with a pain in her neck and lumbar spine; she had experienced pain for quite a while after giving birth. She had a little daughter who was diagnosed with Asperger's Syndrome,[12] which meant she needed a lot of special care from her mother.

She explained her symptoms to me, and we talked about her everyday life and how she took care of her body.

She herself had been diagnosed with a very rare connective tissue disease, so rare I had never heard about it before during my studies. It took me some time to look it up in my pathology books. She was diagnosed as a teenager, and she was on lifelong medicine to keep it under control.

She was told not to have high expectations for her life, and the doctor was sure she wouldn't be able to follow through with a normal college degree.

She told me how she remembered feeling really angry inside all the way to her core. She was furious about being told not to expect too much from life at a time when she felt the world was at her feet, and she thought she was invincible.

This woman decided that NO ONE could tell her what she could and could not do! She made a shift in her consciousness, instead of giving up and feeling defeated.

---

[12] *Asperger's syndrome is* named after the Austrian pediatrician, Hans Asperger, who, in 1944, studied and described children in his practice who lacked nonverbal communication skills, demonstrated limited empathy with their peers, and were physically clumsy.

Chapter 2: Our Own Worst Enemy

In the following years, she graduated from college and even went to university and became a very successful lawyer and a powerful woman.

After hearing her story, I knew she had a strong mindset, but she had a lot on her plate. She didn't expect to give birth to a special needs child, so when it happened, she didn't get to deal with the emotions surrounding this new life. It is normal to be triggered when things don't turn out the way you expected. It doesn't mean you don't love your child, it just means be aware if you have any suppressed emotions.

I saw her for a couple of months and worked on releasing her stress and tension in her spine and focusing on taking some time for herself without having to take care of her daughter 24/7 by delegating some of the responsibility to her husband, and she ended up feeling amazing in her body again. The connective tissue disease was still there, but it wasn't dominating her life anymore.

She was a great example of a woman who would not be stopped by obstacles and just continued living life on her terms; she didn't base her life on other people's limiting beliefs about her and neither should you. Become aware of what is holding you back, and you are halfway there. Be courageous enough to honestly recognize the feeling you might have about your situation and remember it's okay to get a diagnosis, but screw the prognosis! You create your own life, don't listen to the Debbie downers.

Another woman came to me completely drained. She was very pale and skinny when I first saw her.

The Fear Bucket List

When she told me her story, I knew I had to help her get back in tune with her body and change her focus.

She and her husband had tried for a second child and were thrilled when they finally got their little princess. But something was wrong and the little baby was in and out of the hospital until she was diagnosed with a rare form of infant leukemia.

Nothing could be done and, sadly, she died nine months later, which resulted in the mother going into severe depression, and the husband leaving her in the end.

She didn't feel like going on living after her little baby was taken away from her. She was afraid of allowing herself to be happy, when something this terrible had happened to her little girl. The trauma had created a lot of fear in her mind, and it was holding her back from living her life.

When I saw her the first time, the loss of her baby girl was still affecting her whole being. It was like a dark cloud surrounding her body.

It had been a year since her baby died, and she was still sad as ever.

I began working on her nervous system very slowly and gently, loosening up her spinal nerves and muscle tension. We also worked a lot on letting go of her fears and accepting what had happened.

She cried a lot the first couple of times, whenever I unblocked her physical tensions. Usually, when I start loosening up the physical tension, the emotional trauma gets released in the form of crying.

After a couple of months with regular treatments, she finally started to get her old personality back. She was ready to let go of the trauma and move on.

She started work again as a schoolteacher and focused on helping the children, and she was more present with her son, whom she had been neglecting throughout her long mourning period.

She even thought about dating again and, for the first time, I saw her beautiful smile and what a smile she had!

It was amazing to witness her transformation of healing, and I am very grateful to this day to have been able to help her along the way.

This is another example of how powerful your emotions can be and how they can affect your whole body. It proves that no matter what happens to you, there is a way to feel better. No matter how dark and unfair it seems, there is light at the end of the tunnel, and you are the only one who can decide what you are going to do with your life.

So, if you have experienced a trauma in your life and are walking around with unexplainable physical symptoms, have it checked and start working on loosening up your body. Release the tension in your body, and your emotions will follow. Fear is just another emotion in your body that, if not addressed, could hold you back.

Chapter 3:
How Fear Can Affect Our Health

"How you feel in any given moment in time is really the result of the meaning that you've given to that experience."

Anthony Robbins

I have felt in my own body how the accumulated fear and emotions from an old trauma can create an unbalance in my body.

I had just made a bold decision to move away from my friends and family in Denmark to start over and try my luck on the other side of the world, in a culture I had never experienced before—Hong Kong. I had met a very nice man who invited me to stay with him, so I decided to go for it and see where this would take me.

I packed my bags and went on a thirteen-hour one-way flight to Hong Kong ("Asia's New York"), the financial center of the world.

The Fear Bucket List

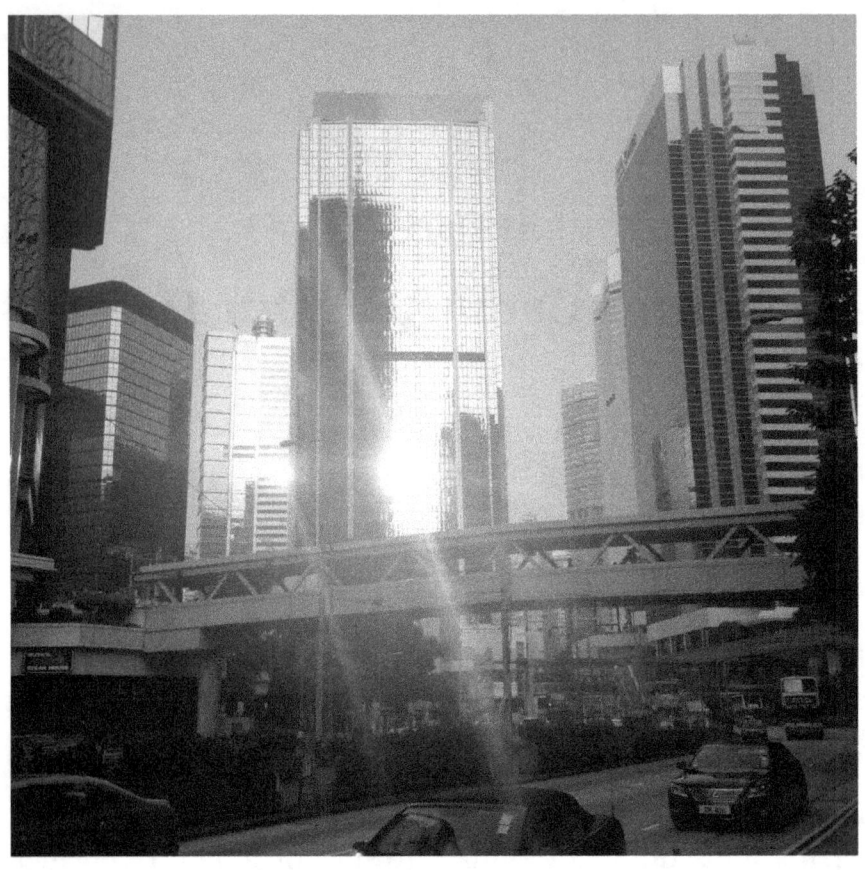

Hong Kong

I didn't plan a return date, which I remember surprised a lot of my friends. But, for me, it felt right. In order for me to focus and be present in the moment, I had to leave the past behind.

I spent the first six months exploring the city, trying to find my way around. I met new like-minded friends, and I was really well received. I visited all the sights and museums and just took in the city.

Chapter 3: How Fear Can Affect Our Health

Hong Kong was very different from my normal life back in Denmark, where working and paying off my loans was a priority; actually, it was like being on a different planet. The buildings were so tall. There were so many people on the streets of varying nationalities, many different languages, and a subtropical climate. It was overwhelming.

I travelled a lot around Asia during that time to Japan, Thailand, and Singapore, and I had many great experiences in a short period of time. But I have always been quite energetic so, when I started sleeping twelve hours a day and feeling nauseous in the morning, I figured something might not be right.

I knew I had had a busy year with ups and downs, including a very bad break up and losing my company as a result of it. I knew I had been losing my hair and feeling very stressed, but my body just kept going, and I didn't want to let my new patients down. I forgot my own preaching about taking care of oneself in order to be there for others.

I knew in my heart that I needed some time off—that's why I flew to Hong Kong in the first place—in order to recover, start over, and take care of myself and fill my body with energy and love again.

I knew this process could take some time, so I started to worry a little bit when I felt more and more tired after six months.

I went to see a local lady doctor and had some routine tests done. At first, they thought I was pregnant because of my nausea symptoms, and I felt quite surprised and happy, but

The Fear Bucket List

the feeling was turned into fear when the test results came back diagnosing me with pre-cervical cancer. I was shocked!

I felt personally how the body and mind are connected. How important it is to be in balance emotionally, in order to be healthy. I was being given a chance to practice on myself, and prove what I had been teaching others.

Of all the fears in my life, cancer probably beats them all!

This was the first real warning I had received in my life, other than severe migraines, telling me how important it was to quickly get back in balance.

Me, the healthy wellness chiropractor and lifestyle coach, I couldn't believe it, but deep inside I knew the reason. I knew everyone has inactive cancer cells in the body, but what can trigger it is a pattern of deep resentment that is held for a long time. It had taken more of my energy than I thought, getting over the shock of losing my business and my relationship.

I was diagnosed on a Friday; they called me while I was in the subway on my way back from IKEA. I had been buying some Scandinavian furniture for the apartment to make me feel at home, and I was completely caught off guard when I received the phone call. I remember hanging up and just letting go of all my bags onto the floor. I was just standing there all alone not knowing what to do. It was like all the sounds had disappeared and everything turned into slow motion. I felt so empty inside and in shock.

The doctor didn't want to risk it developing or spreading further, so they urged me to have surgery five days later. I

Chapter 3: How Fear Can Affect Our Health

had never had surgery before, and I remember the night before the surgery thinking *Tomorrow I will be facing two fears—fear of needles and fear of dying while under a general anesthetic.*

I must have been in the hospital for only half an hour when the nurse wanted to take a blood test. I decided to just relax and look the other way. Every time I have my blood drawn, I get less and less scared of it.

When I was in chiropractor school, we had to practice drawing blood on each other and, needless to say, it didn't make me a fan. Later on, I would faint whenever I saw a needle, or had a blood test, so it was a bit of an obstacle for me. But, because I refused to let the fear win and changed my mindset, I actually had a good experience this time. I barely felt it, and I didn't faint.

I remember lying in the hospital bed waiting for the anesthesiologist to arrive to put me under. I was feeling nervous, because I had never been under a general anesthetic before, so I didn't know how I would react to it. Again, my disadvantage was knowing all the possible side effects, which didn't make it any easier. I decided to relax and think positive and, before I knew it, I was waking up.

I remember getting a phone call from my doctor a couple of days later, giving me the green light. I was completely cleared, the surgery had been successful, and there were no bad cells left.

The happiness I felt was indescribable. It made me feel so grateful for life, and I appreciated it even more. But it also made me even more aware of how important the body-mind balance is to us humans.

Self-healing exercise

I used this exercise in the following days to heal my body after the surgery.

Find a quiet spot. Imagine you are breathing in a white light and direct it to the part of your body where you are experiencing pain, let it cradle the area with love, then exhale the pain imagining a dark cloud and let go.

Repeat this at least three times out loud:

"*Even though I have this (pain), I completely accept and love myself.*"

The greatest guru is your own experience in this life.

To become more aware, ask yourself questions like "What is this pain telling me?"

"What message am I not seeing?"

"Why is this happening today? What is the lesson I need to learn from this?"

Do this instead of blaming yourself or others.

PART II – From the Beginning

"That which does not kill us makes us stronger."

Friedrich Nietzsche

Chapter 4:
Learning How to Swim the Frogman Way

I had a very happy childhood. I grew up in Copenhagen, Denmark, in 'Nyboder' (the yellow naval barracks built by Christian IV in 1631), because my father worked for the Danish Frogman Corps.[13]

My mum was seventeen years younger than my father and worked in a bank, which sometimes meant long hours. Often the neighbor, a female corrections officer, would look after me and my younger sister, or I would look after the both of us. Sometimes my dad would be there, when my mum was on an evening course further educating herself, in order to move up the ranks, and we would usually have pancakes for dinner, which was a big hit.

I walked my sister to school every day from the age of seven. Denmark was a safe place to grow up and, although we

---

[13] *Danish Frogman Corps: an elite counter-terrorism special forces of the Royal Danish Navy equivalent to Navy SEALS or The British Special Boat Service (SBS).*

didn't have much, we had enough. Our family of four started out in a tiny apartment, where we shared a toilet in the hallway with another family, and we had no shower. It was always freezing in the wintertime, because none of the houses were insulated properly, and in the summer American tourists would come to Copenhagen on big cruise ships and walk around Nyboder and look in through our windows, thinking it was a museum or something.

I remember that my father had his shotgun hanging in the wardrobe behind the front door, and whenever he returned from a mission, he would bring it out to shoot the big rats running around in our little backyard from the first floor window. I liked watching him load the gun, but I always hoped he would miss the rats.

To decompress from reality, he kept small rainbow-colored tropical birds in a special room, and he would sit in this room for hours just watching the birds. He loved animals, and quite often he would take me and my sister out to the forest to listen to the birds. Whoever guessed the most birds won. I really looked up to him. He was the fiercest man I knew, and all I wanted was to make him proud. Whenever my father was promoted, we would move to a bigger apartment, and eventually we moved into a full house with the luxury of a shower and a bathtub.

Every weekend and holiday, we would leave Copenhagen and take our rescue Doberman, Santa, and drive to our summerhouse on the other side of the island. It was built in the seventies by my father in solid wood and had a huge fireplace. My happiest memories are from that

Chapter 4: Learning How to Swim the Frogman Way

summerhouse, and I remember really enjoying getting out of the city and into nature.

The summerhouse was surrounded by a big beautiful lush garden supplying us with fresh vegetables, fruits, and berries. I enjoyed picking berries with my sister and watching my mother turn them into delicious jam.

Early in the morning, my father would wake me up and take me out in his little orange rowing boat to catch salmon. I loved sitting in the front of the boat while he rowed, just watching the water flow by and enjoying the silence and the time alone just him and me.

My mother would be in the kitchen making fresh coffee and baking bread and cakes ready for our return. She always made everything from scratch and put all her love into it. We all enjoyed the smell of freshly baked bread wafting through the house and, whenever we got tired of eating salmon, he would trade the fish for turkey at the local farm.

My sister and I spent hours playing outside every day. When the summer thunderstorms came, we would run out on the wet grass and dance naked in the pouring rain. It was the happiest time of my life; I felt so free, safe, and loved.

I remember the summer, just before starting my first year of school and before anything happened to me, I was five years old, and my father decided to teach me how to swim. We walked down to the beach, where an old wooden bridge led out about twenty meters into the cold Scandinavian water. The bridge had two metal ladders, one leading down to the shallow water and one leading to the deeper water.

The Fear Bucket List

After explaining the basic principles of avoiding to inhale under water and kicking my arms and legs, he threw me right in! Talk about facing your fears head on and diving right in—literally!

I remember being scared of touching the bottom, because I didn't like crabs, so I kicked and kicked and stayed afloat on the surface. The water was quite cold, and my body was still in shock from landing in it. Instinctively, I wanted to get back to the ladder closest to me, but my father told me to try to swim to the next one further in. While keeping an eye on me and making sure I was safe, he yelled commands and directions, like I was one of his frogman recruits and, as a result, I ended up swimming all the way to the second ladder.

He had this amazing ability to push me beyond my limits in a good way and never give up. He taught me that *sometimes the very things you don't like are the things you need to go beyond.* He empowered me with lessons like this throughout my childhood. He also taught me how to shoot, throw a hand grenade and survive in the forest like Bear Grylls.

I think a lot of my strength comes from my father, and I've used that strength many times throughout my life when things seemed impossible, or I wanted to give up. I never forgot my foundation, and I always remember my childhood with a smile on my face. I'm sure it also played a part in how I handled everything later on in life. The fact that I knew I was loved by my parents gave me an advantage. Not everyone is lucky enough to have this unfortunately. I know everybody's journey is different.

Chapter 5:
When Everything Changed – The Effects of Sexual Abuse

"If you use your wounds to grow and learn, you don't have to stay a victim."

Oprah Winfrey

I was only six years old when my fifteen-year-old cousin sexually abused me.

Up until that day, I had been a happy, outgoing girl who loved dressing up and putting on a show for anyone who would watch me. I liked to laugh and be around other children. I really loved my life, my family, and playing in nature. I had a sense of self-worth and felt special inside.

That was all taken away from me one afternoon, while I was visiting family in Jutland, Denmark.

Both my parents had moved to Copenhagen as teenagers, but the rest of their family had stayed behind, in northern Jutland, as far away from Copenhagen as possible (about a four-hour drive). Usually, I loved going there to visit my grandmother, because we shared a very special bond. We would stay up late and watch ice skating on TV.

One day, my parents, little sister, and I, were visiting one of my uncles, and the grownups were spending time together in the living room, while we, my cousins, and their friends, were running around the neighborhood. There was a great age gap between us all. Some were a few years older, some were teenagers, and some were young adults, but me and my sister were the youngest.

Usually, my older cousin would tease my sister and me and throw firecrackers at us, but he targeted me more than anyone. I didn't know why at the time, and I thought he was just being silly. On this particular day, he got me separated from the others, and that is when the sexual abuse happened.

I will spare you and not go into details here, as my book is about so much more than dwelling in the past, plus I believe that my subconscious mind shut down this memory on purpose and repressed it. All I remember is a football field and being forced to do things that felt very uncomfortable. This is very normal when you experience something traumatic. I just want you to get a sense of why I started being afraid and lost my self-confidence in the first place.

After this incident, he told me that if I said anything to anyone, he would do the same to my sister, so I decided to keep my mouth shut in order to protect her. I had no clue about sexuality at that age; all I remember was feeling very uncomfortable during the experience and dirty and ashamed afterwards, like it was my fault. I felt that there

Chapter 5: When Everything Changed

must be something wrong with me, if he would choose to do something like that to me. I concluded that I must be a very bad person to deserve something so horrible.

Needless to say, I stopped enjoying my visits to Jutland after that, but until my grandmother died of a stroke four years later, I had to go there every year. I missed my grandmother like crazy, but I was relieved that I didn't have to see my cousin's face ever again.

I kept my secret hidden from those closest to me for fifteen years. At first, I kept silent to protect my younger sister but, later on, I realized how important it was for me to keep it a secret from my parents, especially my father, who was a special force marine and had joined the navy as a young man in order to protect his family.

I was convinced that if he ever discovered the truth, he would make my cousin disappear for what he had done to his little girl. I was scared my father would be sent to prison, and I really didn't want to lose him.

I have always been very close to my father. He's a very good man, so keeping the truth from him was probably the hardest thing I ever did. In my own way, I felt like I had to, in order to keep him in my life, but I also wanted to protect him. If he learned the truth, he would blame himself for not being able to protect his daughter from an enemy so close to home. He would be devastated.

Throughout my upbringing, my father would look at me and say, "Kamilla, just be yourself!" It hurt me so deeply that I wasn't able to explain to him why I couldn't. He obviously sensed that I was not being one hundred percent myself anymore and wondered why his little girl had changed.

I wasn't relaxed anymore. I became more introverted and stopped performing in front of people. I developed a mask personality disguising who I really was, hiding my emotions in order to cope with the pressure of keeping my secret. It slowly developed into an emotional prison. Whenever I felt sad, I would think of a beautiful field of flowers or little puppies in order to stop myself from crying, resulting in a constant feeling of a lump in my throat, a feeling of being choked. I made sure no one got too close to me, buried my nose in books, focused on sports, and secretly hated all boys.

All I wanted was to tell my father the real reason why I had changed. I had so many chances, but I never did.

The abuse happened around the same time I started school and had to deal with a lot of new children. I was so scared that if anyone came too close to me and really got to know me, they would find out the truth. I feared that if the kids at school knew, they wouldn't like me, and they would look at me differently, or they would think I was a disgusting, dirty person.

I felt like my spirit had been broken, like I wasn't really there. It was like I grew up in an instant. I developed an introverted personality and suffered from low self-esteem, self-doubt, and a critical attitude towards myself and my body, never really feeling good enough or worthy. I tried to please others and became obsessed with controlling everything I did. I needed to know what people thought about me at all times in order to be one step ahead. I would sometimes have intense bursts of anger and hatred triggered by random things, like watching a movie or the news where sexual abuse was mentioned.

EFFECTS OF THE ABUSE

The little girl inside me disappeared, and so did the need for attention. I lost my childhood in an instant and started worrying about what other people thought about me. I stopped dancing ballet and became more masculine, in order to protect myself, and started focusing on athletics after school in order to keep my mind busy. In my teenage years, I hid my body in oversized hoodies and baggy pants, because I didn't want anyone looking at my body.

I wanted to please people and fit into the grownup world. I found it difficult listening to my heart, because I was *afraid* to stand out. I spent all my days reading and getting good grades, so I had the option of going to the best universities when the time came. I forgot to have fun and took life very seriously. I didn't drink like all the other students. The only place I really enjoyed being was at the athletics stadium where I could concentrate on sports to keep myself sane.

I used my pain and anger to focus on athletics. My favorite discipline was long jump and high jump, but I also loved sprinting as fast as I could. In those moments of competition, I forgot about everything else. I slowly trained to become a heptathlete—doing seven different activities during a competition.

The Fear Bucket List

I made the stadium my sanctuary because it gave me strength.

In the beginning, it felt like everyone ran faster than me, jumped higher than me, and jumped further than me, but instead of feeling like a failure, it created a fire inside of me to improve my technique more and more and train even harder, until I eventually had the feeling of being the best at something.

This feeling helped me to go on. The encouragement from my coaches also really helped me through this time in my life. It was a really nice feeling to have someone rooting for me and my results and, before I knew it, I was the best in my year group, and I kept beating my own personal records again and again.

My coach sent me to a chiropractor at the age of thirteen, and I had my spine aligned for the first time, which helped me to run faster and jump higher, because all of a sudden I felt more open in my lumbar spine and hips. It was a great shift in my body awareness. I thought it was the coolest thing ever that this guy with nothing but his hands helped me get an edge on my competitors, and it sparked my later path into chiropractic.

I started loving what I was doing, because athletics helped me gain confidence, and it provided a place where I felt safe. Throughout my teenage years, that's what kept me sane. The second I stepped into the stadium, I felt alive, like I owned that place. "The athlete" was my favorite persona, because it was the only part of my life where I felt like I knew what I was doing. The rest of the time, I felt pretty lost.

Chapter 5: When Everything Changed

I remember that every time I threw my javelin, I imagined my cousin at the end of it. It helped me to release my hatred towards him, but my anger kept resurfacing.

I was seventeen years old in my senior year of high school, and I was sure I was the last virgin left in my year. I had two sexual encounters that year. The first one was with a boy two years my junior who lived next door to my best friend. He was a virgin too, and I quickly zoomed in on him as my perfect 'first time'. I figured since both of us were inexperienced, it wouldn't be too embarrassing. I just wanted to get it over with and know what everyone was talking about.

My second encounter was with a much older guy from Togo. I don't remember where I met him, but I was fascinated by his six feet four inches and beautiful dark skin. He told me he had been in the Foreign Legion back in his home country before coming to Denmark. So, my first impression was that he must be a good guy like my father fighting for his country. He was fluent in French and worked out all the time.

I kept our meetings secret, because I wasn't sure how my parents would react to him. At first, he was very nice to me. He taught me French and worked out with me between athletics practice and school. I would sneak out and meet him sometimes at his place, and it was all very interesting until one day he was at my house, when nobody was home.

He started by wanting to take photos of me, which I found a bit odd. It made me quite uncomfortable, but I tried not to show it. I didn't want to be the boring young girl. But then

The Fear Bucket List

he suddenly grabbed me, put my hands behind my back, and held me down. He scared me, and I told him to please stop, but he didn't. He wanted what he wanted, and he wanted it his way—fully aware that no one could hear me scream.

Afterwards he just left me crying on the bed. I remember feeling a lot of physical pain and then I started thinking, what if he gave me a disease? I knew I couldn't tell my parents, because it was just too humiliating. I had let him in. I trusted him, and I felt completely ashamed.

The next day I went to see a doctor and asked for an HIV test. I didn't tell him why, and he just asked me how recently I had been sexually active. When I replied yesterday, he laughed and told me I had to wait for three months to be tested to see if the virus was present, which, in my case, was completely absurd as I was a "nice young woman." He had no idea why I was so concerned. He didn't know I had just been raped, by a thirty four year old guy from West Africa.

Shortly after the rape, I graduated high school and left my athletics career behind to everyone's surprise. I was on top of my sports career and was about to change into the serious leagues, like my half-brother before me, but I just couldn't handle it all. I needed to get away. So, when my father's best friend gave me a graduation present, a ticket to Havana, Cuba, where he was doing some business at the time, I left right away.

I actually had a great time on Cuba, and I even learned photography from a Canadian friend of his. The creativity took my mind off the rape, and I started to feel alive again. I

Chapter 5: When Everything Changed

also started drinking rum, which was very unlike me, because when I was training for the athletics, I wasn't allowed to drink. But, now that I had turned eighteen, I could decide on my own. I discovered how the alcohol would make me forget everything for a while, and I could actually have fun and let loose for a little without worrying what other people thought about me. My self-awareness vanished, and I became a different person.

When I returned home from Cuba, my parents thought it would be a good idea for me to apply for university. In order to get into a chiropractor school, I needed some experience with people, so I travelled to England first and did some work in a nursing home.

In university, once again, I was buried in books, but this time I was partying and drinking with my fellow students and doing modeling jobs to pay for my books and rent. I convinced myself I needed the escape, and my behavior became more and more selfish and erratic.

I wasn't satisfied in any relationship until I started a '50 Shades Of Grey' relationship with an older guy. I craved being dominated and humiliated, which I found quite paradoxical and a bit embarrassing to admit after the rape. I also thought something was seriously wrong with me. I had numerous relationships and sexual encounters in my twenties. I think I was trying to punish my own body just to feel something, anything. I also experimented with drugs, which was easily accessible in the modeling world.

In the back of my mind, fear was controlling my life. I was scared of losing my parents, scared of people not liking me, scared I wasn't good enough, scared of spiders, scared of heights, scared of people knowing who I really was, and I was scared of telling the truth about how I felt.

It felt very restricted, like an invisible cage. It was holding me back in so many ways and made me feel alone. It took me many years to start working on my fears and abuse, and it didn't happen overnight.

I wasn't born fearful, but I slowly adapted to my surroundings and let the fear take over.

***

Most people lose their innocence in one way or the other. I lost mine on a football field at the age of six and again at the age of seventeen in my own home.

THE TURNING POINT – WHEN I FINALLY TOLD SOMEONE

I must have been around twenty-one years old and on year two of university, when I went to Damascus, Syria, with my boyfriend and his family for a wedding. It was a completely different world from what I was used to. We weren't allowed to hold hands or kiss in public. I had to cover up my hair and ankles to avoid being harassed on the street.

I remember at the wedding how the men and women were separated right after the ceremony. The men would sit on the roof and smoke shisha while the women were downstairs. All the women arrived at the wedding covered

Chapter 5: When Everything Changed

up. All you could see was their black painted eyes peeping out.

The main subject of conversation was marriage. It was like going back to the middle ages. They couldn't understand why I wasn't married yet and why I was studying instead of having children. I decided just to keep my thoughts to myself, as I was a guest, and it really wasn't my business how they lived their lives. But it hurt me deep inside seeing them focus on things like this and not on education for themselves.

The second the men left the room to go upstairs, an oriental remix of Usher was put on the stereo, and the women took off their head covers and a black garment called an *abayah* that covered them from shoulders to feet, leaving behind a big pile of black material on the floor. All of a sudden, I was the most covered-up girl in the room, as they were now wearing tiny cocktail dresses and stilettos and dancing around in a circle, while the elder women were sitting on chairs observing who had the longest hair, best moves, and widest hips. Apparently, weddings were a way for the mothers of the men to pick out a future wife for their son. It reminded me a bit of a cattle market.

The next day we went on a sightseeing trip around Damascus visiting the market and some mosques. It was really hot outside, and I felt like melting in the desert sun. When we arrived at the entrance of one of the mosques, the guard told me to wear an abayah and another head cover on top of my clothing before entering. I understood that there was nothing I could do to protest, so I just put it on and walked in with sweat dripping from my head.

The Fear Bucket List

Inside the mosque, my boyfriend kept laughing at me. He wanted to take pictures of me, because I looked like a penguin. He just kept laughing and coming at me with his camera, so I told him to please just leave me alone. He didn't listen and kept agitating me until I finally completely freaked out in the middle of the mosque in front of everyone in his family and other guests there.

Inside of me, I just couldn't handle the way the women were suppressed and had to cover up at all times. Coming from a culture and a world where women are equal and very well educated, it just triggered me so much, that I found myself screaming out loud followed by breaking down in unstoppable tears. They had to escort me out of there in order for me not to get arrested. This was the first time I had really cried and let it all out. It was like the final drop made the glass overflow.

Later that night I had to apologize to the whole family for my behavior and excused myself with lying about being emotional because of PMS.[14]

I realize now that my reaction was an entirely normal reaction in humans who have suffered some sort of trauma, sexual or otherwise.[15] It is not unusual to experience sudden mood swings or even rage. The brain is not developed enough at the age of six to be able to process the experience or the emotions to go along with it. In my early twenties, I was still walking around with the consciousness of a six-

---

[14] *PMS: Premenstrual syndrome, common symptoms are irritability and mood changes.*
[15] *www.stopitnow.org*

Chapter 5: When Everything Changed

year-old girl who felt responsible and guilty for putting myself in a situation where sexual abuse could happen.

Later that night my boyfriend asked me if it was okay for his father to come to talk to me in our hotel room. He obviously hadn't bought my story about freaking out because of PMS and he encouraged me to speak out about why I had so much anger inside. For the first time ever, I talked about what happened to me as a child and he made me promise to tell my parents when I returned home. Afterwards I fell in a deep sleep, and my body relaxed a little more than usual.

I'll never forget the look on my father's face when I told him. He just started crying—my dad, the super hero special forces marine, balling his eyes out. He admitted that he had had his suspicions back when I was a little girl, because I changed all of a sudden. He even remembered asking me about it, but I had looked him straight in the eyes and denied it, so he just left it alone.

My mum was crying too. She felt bad, because it was someone from her family who had abused me. She told me she was happy that she had cut off contact with her brother and his family after their mother died, so I didn't have to see them again. She also told me that her brother had been a real bastard towards his son and that he probably had a very hard upbringing. It made me feel a little sorry for my abuser for the first time, thinking about him as a human being who might even have been abused himself.

Chapter 6:
Date with Destiny

"You are NOT your story!"

Anthony Robbins

Besides my random anger attacks, I suffered from low self-esteem and a distorted view of my body. Even though I was working regularly as a model, I felt awkward and not pretty at all. I was told to lose weight over and over again, even though I was already too skinny.

For a young woman, it can be really hard to be in that business, where constant critique is an everyday thing. Unfortunately, it also fed my need to punish my body, by starving myself and later throwing up after eating too much, feeling guilty that I had consumed too many calories. Many of my fellow model friends ended up addicted to drugs and struggled with eating disorders long after their modeling career ended.

I finally finished my studies at age twenty-five and landed a chiropractor job in a private clinic in Copenhagen.

The Fear Bucket List

On the outside, everything looked normal, but I kept hitting a wall. Several relationships had gone down the drain, and I knew something drastic had to be done, in order to change my life ... I just didn't know what yet. I realized my fear was getting in the way of living a productive and happy life.

I was so tired of being angry, not trusting anyone, doubting myself, and pretending to be someone else. I knew I had a problem. I knew I had a pattern of feeling sorry for myself, not taking responsibility, and playing the victim in different situations. I had enough, so I packed my bags.

The journey I decided to go on was to a self-help course with Anthony Robbins. Pandora's box had been opened, and I knew I needed to take my self-healing to the next level, so when I heard about a six-day course called "Date With Destiny," I maxed out my credit card and travelled to Palm Springs.

***

Notebook entry

I guess this is the point of no return. I'm sitting in the back of this Boeing 747 looking at the wings carrying me to the United States of America. It's still daylight outside, the sky is bright blue, and the moon is almost full, hovering above the sea of clouds. It's December and already very cold in Denmark. I don't mind leaving for a warmer climate—destination Palm Springs!

I don't know what is waiting for me over the next couple of days, but I know this is the right time to explore my inner

Chapter 6: Date with Destiny

self ... after so many years of secrets ... I know this, because I feel excited and a little bit scared at the same time of what I might learn. I know it's only my ego trying to scare me away from taking this journey. But this journey has already begun. There's no turning back now, and I am ready.

***

I was really scared when I entered the seminar room on the first day, everyone was dancing on the chairs, and loud music was playing in the background. People were hugging and high-fiving each other for no apparent reason. I found the whole scenario a bit odd and started doubting my decision to attend the event. It was freezing cold, so I had to go back to my room to get my jacket. On the way to my room, I realized that maybe I was the one being odd for not participating in whatever it was everyone was doing, after all, I had paid a lot of money and come all this way.

When I returned, I decided to stand on a chair like everyone else and slowly started clapping my hands and shaking my hips side to side (in a very controlled way—I didn't want to give anyone the wrong impression). I was still so concerned with what other people thought about me.

On day two, we were split up into smaller groups, and we had to pair-up with a buddy. I was too shy to pick anyone so I just waited until someone came over and started talking to me. On the following days, we would share our inner thoughts, do exercises together and support each other, not only in the buddy pairs but also in the smaller group setting.

The Fear Bucket List

I especially remember one episode where the senior coach paired me up with a forty-year-old African-American man. She had obviously read my file. Before entering "Date with Destiny" everyone fills out a questionnaire with details about their personal story. I had mentioned the rape as a teenager and the senior coach now wanted me to stand in front of this stranger and look him in the eyes without breaking eye contact.

At first, I refused and started shaking and crying. I wanted to run away. I didn't want to stand near him, let alone look him in the eyes. It felt too frightening to me after my bad experience. But she insisted and told the guy to just be the space that I needed to heal.

He just stood there, and I finally gathered all my courage and looked him in the eyes. It didn't take long before I started crying, but after a while, I started feeling the calmness and love directed at me, and my body relaxed more and more, until I felt no resentment towards him. We finished off the exercise with a big bear hug and went back to the seminar hall to do some more dancing.

Tony taught me a lot of lessons that week including being less self-conscious by taking me out of my comfort zone, and because I was in a peak state, it was easier to reprogram my body and mind in order to move forward in my life. It was the beginning of my transformation.

One of the lessons was *"See it as it is, not worse than it is. See it better than it is, then make it the way you see it."*

Chapter 6: Date with Destiny

I had never heard anything like this before, and I was reminded of my own habits of always making the worst assumptions about people and situations.

The most important lesson of the entire week was **_"You are NOT your story!"_** He told me to recognize that the life you live right now is because of YOU, not your family, not your boyfriend, not your economy, but YOU. You need to take responsibility for your own life and make the commitment to change your path if you are not satisfied. *The past cannot be changed. You are not your story. Accept it. Trust that there is a higher purpose.*

I decided right there and then that I was going to change my life and start taking responsibility and not be a victim anymore.

Just think about that for a minute ... what does that even mean? *You are NOT your story* ... for me it meant the beginning of a release from the secret I had been carrying around for years. I had already done the hard part, which for me was finally telling my parents about my abuse. Now was the time to step it up a notch and continue the journey I had started.

It was a hard week for me emotionally, and, honestly, I just wanted to leave several times ... I was too scared of what I might find if I dug deep enough. And it seemed easier to just pick up and leave, but I didn't. I stayed even though I was feeling nauseous and scared.

I realized that I had been focusing on myself all these years and become a victim, trapped in my past.

Many people in the room had experienced much worse things than I had, and it put things in perspective.

I know this sounds harsh, but it doesn't matter what happened to you, all that matters is HOW you decide to live your life. Are you going to blame people and have anger in your heart, or are you going to overcome it by stepping out of the victim role and use your wounds to grow and learn? It's all about your mindset.

I worked a lot on my emotions and my fears that week, by opening up and talking about my experiences again and again in the group, until I couldn't cry anymore. During an exercise of connecting to my heart, guided by Tony Robbins, I visualized my cousin in front of me and forgave him for what he had done to me. I saw him as a little boy being yelled at by his father and shamed by him, and it released a lot of old hatred and anger. I also saw myself first as a little girl, then as a teenager, and then as a young adult and forgave myself for punishing my body all these years. This whole process lasted about forty-five minutes and, by the end of it, I felt like a weight had been lifted off my shoulders.

This event inspired me to begin writing my book, as I needed a higher meaning with what had happened to me. In that moment, I realized I wouldn't change a thing.

I know that who I am today is because of the accumulated events of my life and, instead of being a victim, I feel empowered to still be here and making a difference in the world.

Chapter 6: Date with Destiny

When I came back from Palm Springs, I focused more on being aware of my underlying thoughts. They didn't just disappear. It was a process, but I was aware of them and started questioning my inner dialog. I made a list of all my good sides and my awesomeness factor, and I read it to myself every morning.

I also started a gratitude journal and appreciated the little wins I had, like a patient thanking me for really listening to them, or being myself around others, or saying no to things that weren't aligned with my inner truth. I started doing things that made me happy like going on meditation retreats alone to emerge myself in my inner world, a world I was slowly starting to appreciate instead of being afraid of it.

I also had a personal coach for about a year following-up on me, which really helped me be accountable. She helped me put down some goals that I wanted to achieve and also worked on my self-love and life purpose. I would later go on and become a certified Tony Robbins Strategic Intervention Coach myself in order to help others the way I was helped.

PART III – In the Footsteps of the Initiates

Chapter 7:
Egypt

Following my "Date with Destiny" adventure, I became more and more interested in my inner world through meditation and spirituality. I started reading a lot of spiritual books in order to find a meaning of it all. I had a couple of spiritual teachers along the way including a Buddhist monk from Ladakh, a Reiki master, a Mayan Elder, and a meditation teacher.

Ever since my mother's best friend passed away from AIDS and left me his book collection, I had been fascinated by old civilizations like the Mayans and the Egyptians and what they could teach us about the world and ourselves. According to the Egyptians, the heart is the source of human wisdom, the center of the soul and the personality, not the brain. They understood that we are not our brain and body, and we create our own reality. Everything in life runs in cycles, and we continually develop our consciousness until we are done on this Earth school.

The Fear Bucket List

They performed many initiation rituals in the Mayan temples in Mexico and in the Egyptian temples in ancient Egypt.

I decided to go on a spiritual pilgrimage of self-healing as a way to get to know my inner self better and get rid of my remaining fears. I knew the key to a happy and fulfilling life was through facing my fears. I had read that facing fears was the way the Egyptians ascended to a higher consciousness, and that's when I had the idea of creating my own personal Fear Bucket List. I didn't just want to live a normal life; I wanted a life of bliss. I was twenty-eight when I started my Fear Bucket List, and I'm still facing fears every single day.

The Egyptians believed that the spirit left the body at death. When the body resurrected, the spirit would return to the body, which was why it was so important for them to preserve it.

This was done by an embalming process. The priest was in charge of this and started by cleaning the body with water from the Nile, and then the brain was removed by leading a bronze hook up the nose and pulling it out. Then a resin solution was pumped into the skull to prevent bacteria from forming. *They believed the brain was insignificant because all thinking was done with the heart. The heart was the core of a person, the seat of emotion, so they left it in the body*. This was very similar to the Mayan beliefs about the importance of the heart.

The lungs, stomach, intestines, and liver were removed with an obsidian blade and put into canopy jars, believed to protect the organs for passage to the next world. The chest cavity was rinsed with palm wine and the body was covered in soda to extract the body fluids. The belly cavity was filled with fabric. After forty days of soda, the body was massaged with oil to soften the skin and give it back its elasticity.

As the last step, the body was wrapped in cotton with gemstones and amulets between the layers and, most importantly, a ruby was placed in front of the heart.

After the embalming process, the pharaoh had to go through a lot of tests and rituals described in *The Book of the Dead*, a book I studied in detail growing up, trying to learn more about this civilization. I always felt a special connection to them.

In the book, it is described how the heart was weighed against the feather of Maat (justice) on a scale. If the heart weighed the most, Osiris would decide whether or not a beast would devour the pharaoh. If he passed the test, he would be allowed to continue on his path in the afterlife towards immortality.

Temple of Hathor

My first stop down the Nile was the **Temple of Hathor.**

At the time I decided to visit Egypt, the country was in turmoil. The military had just overthrown president Mursi and the local people were causing havoc in Cairo. Luckily, I was still allowed to take my trip down the Nile as the last tourist as long as I avoided the Cairo area and flew straight back after.

The Fear Bucket List

Many times before, I had tried to go to Egypt, but for some reason, my trip was cancelled several times because the Foreign Ministry of Denmark advised me not to go there. But, I was determined to follow in the footsteps of the Egyptians and face some of my fears.

I arrived at the site and the temperature was well over forty degrees Celsius in the Egyptian desert.

I was really looking forward to seeing this temple and spending time there, as I was working with pregnant women and babies in my clinic every day. This was a very special temple for me to visit, to channel this ancient wisdom and healing powers.

In the old days, a women's hospital was part of the Hathor Temple and was used to worship the goddess. Here, women would come and get help with fertility and giving birth, which was a dangerous thing back then. There was a holy well here, where the water was said to have healing powers and could make a woman fertile.

I quickly disappeared from the group I was with, to go explore the site and its many colonnades, twisted pathways, side temples, and offering spaces. Suddenly, I bumped into a man in a white tunic with a turban; he looked like a local Bedouin. He asked me to follow him quickly before the guard discovered us. My heart started pounding. I didn't know if this was such a good idea, but he seemed like he really wanted to show me something, so I decided to go with him. I had come all this way after all.

Chapter 7: Egypt

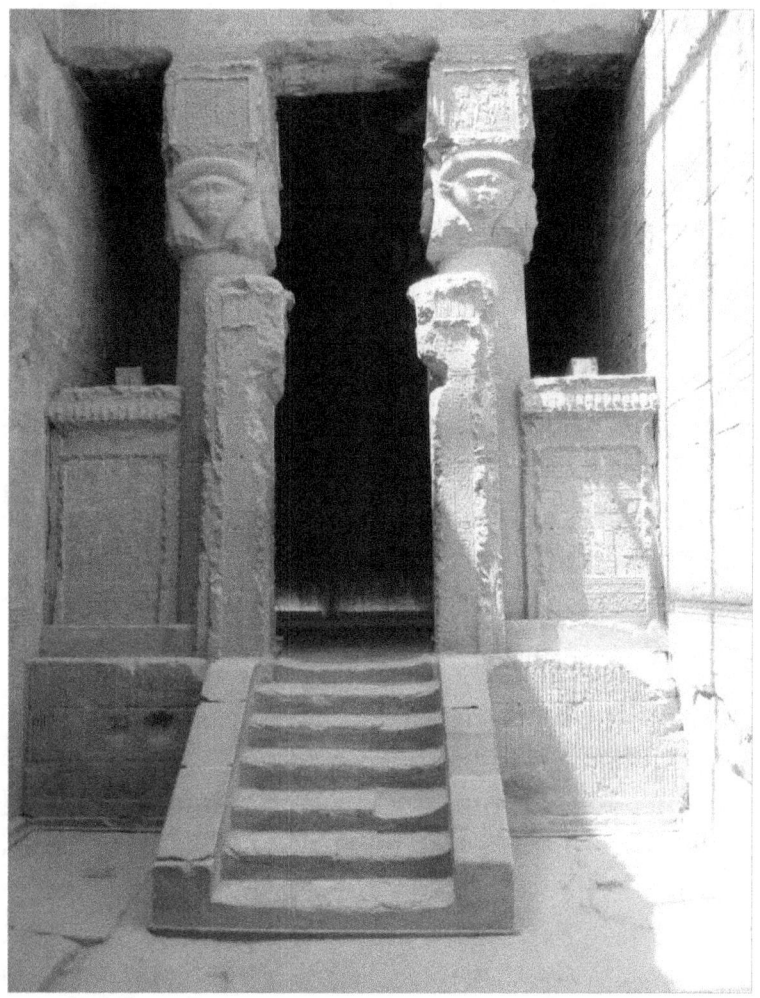

Mini Hathor Temple inside the complex

He led me into the far right side of the temple. In the old days, only the high priestesses were allowed in there in the holiest of all rooms. It looked like a mini Hathor Temple inside the temple itself. He then allowed me to sit in silence and meditate there all by myself. It was almost as if he knew I was coming.

Calmness immediately settled in the room that I had never experienced before. It overwhelmed me with love like a wave. I was not scared or worried anymore, but happy and calm, even a little touched.

The subconscious fear of whether or not it would be safe to be in Egypt at that exact time disappeared, and I felt protected.

The Bedouin was waiting for me at the end of the stairs when I finished my meditation. He led me round and round until we reached a corner of the temple closed off by a net on the floor. He looked around to make sure it was clear, and then lifted the net and pointed down into the dark hole, where a very steep staircase led downwards to what seemed to be a dead end wall.

I slowly crawled down the hole and descended into the dark pathway. When I reached the wall, I could see a small opening in the bottom big enough for me to squeeze underneath to the other side. The pathway took a ninety-degree turn right away, and I turned on my iPhone torch. I could see a long corridor going right and one going left. The hallway was covered with intact beautiful reliefs of Hathor. Unfortunately, it wasn't possible to get a decent picture down there because it was so dark.

In the rest of the temple, Hathor's face had been chiseled away by the Romans, who thought she was some kind of evil spirit. Many of the reliefs were destroyed forever, but in the crypt under the temple, her face was still as beautiful as when it was built in 1500 BCE.

Chapter 7: Egypt

The Bedouin asked my permission and performed a sacred initiation ritual for me, a ritual that was passed down through generations from his ancestors.

Following the ritual, he left me to meditate again in the crypt, this time with my back up against the wall and my hands folded over my chest like the Egyptians were positioned when buried. My phone was turned off, and I just stood there in darkness for a while meditating. The energy from the rocks was very strong. It felt like a different dimension down there, and I felt very close to my ancestors.

After the meditation, I slowly made my way up to the surface again, down the corridor, under the stone wall, and up the steep staircase. A guard was on his way, and I had to hurry up and leave, before he saw anything, as I didn't want to get into trouble.

I finished up in the first little temple where I started and said a little prayer, giving thanks for the energy I had just experienced on this very special day, a day I will never forget.

The Bedouin gave me a warm hug and blessed me with future fertility in the spirit of Hathor.

Walking away from the site, I could feel the tears running down my face. The experience released tons of old blocked energy in my body, and I felt connected to my heart stronger than ever before. I felt how my masculine side just melted away and was replaced by a maternal and feminine feeling

The Fear Bucket List

all the way to my core, a feeling I had never felt before in my life.

To finish off the visit, I had a small cup of mint tea with the guards in the entrance to the temple, to give my respect. They seemed happy here just before Ramadan.

Kom Ombo

Fear of spiders, snakes, and scorpions

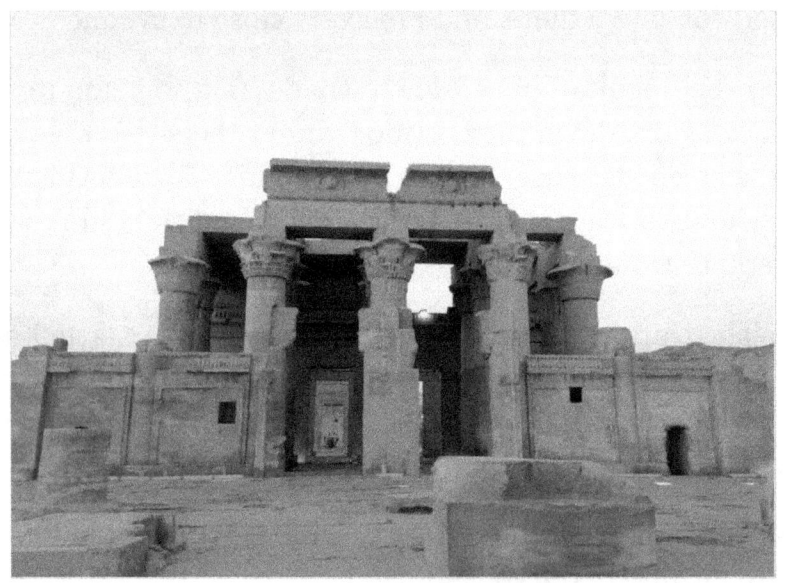

Kom Ombo represents the second chakra—base chakra / sexuality. Here rituals were performed in ancient Egypt, where the initiates would be forced to confront their fears. Some died trying, but the ones who survived became

Chapter 7: Egypt

spiritual leaders and priests or priestesses and served in the temples.

This place also represented balancing the masculine and feminine energy in the form of polarity, which was the basis of sexuality.

Arriving at the temple, I immediately left the group again like last time and started looking around. I was searching for a very special passageway to a crypt, where the ancient Egyptian initiates had to go through, in order to pass the test of the temple.

While searching, I quickly got the attention of another Bedouin and asked him to show me the temple.

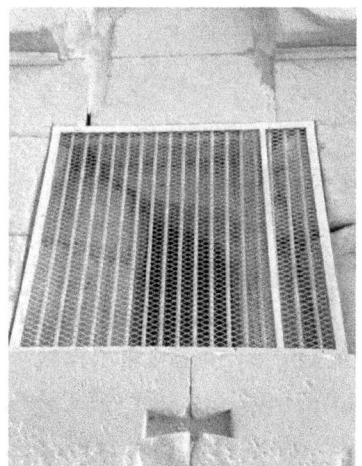

Entrance

After the little tour, I found myself standing right in front of a closed grid on the floor, and I recognized it as the special crypt marked with an hourglass cut into the stone.

The Fear Bucket List

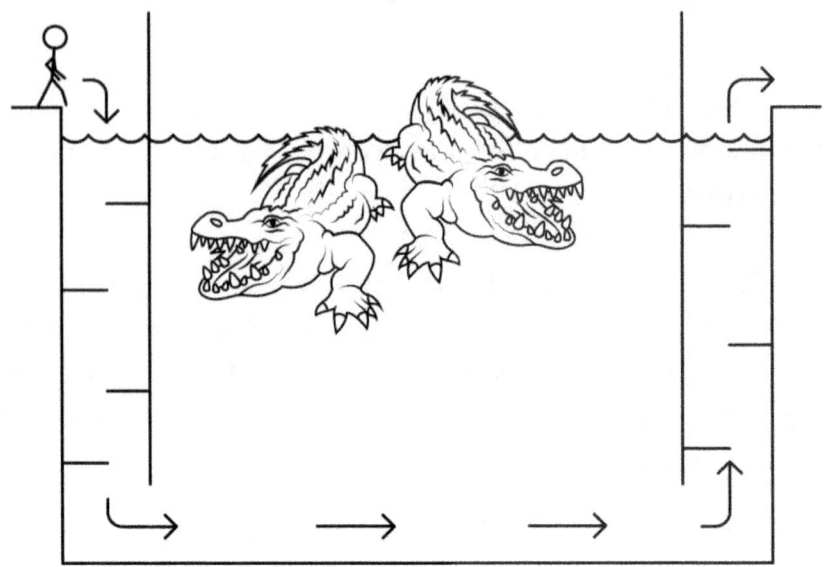

Back then, the initiate had to jump down a very small hole filled with water and was told not to exit at the same place as they entered.

Once the initiate jumped down, he would have to hold his breath and swim downwards until he saw light emanating in front of him. Looking up to the surface, all he could see was black shadows of something moving in the water. He would have to decide whether to swim upwards, like most people did, knowing the shadows were probably crocodiles! But, if he made it to the surface without being attacked, he would be told that he had failed the test. The correct exit was to continue past the obvious light and continue into the dark, where a narrow tunnel led upwards to the surface.

This was definitely the ultimate test of courage, facing your fears of the unknown, drowning, crocodiles and, at the same

Chapter 7: Egypt

time, trusting your intuition. You had to fight the urge to swim upwards at the first chance you got and continue in the dark before ascending, while holding your breath all the way, which would be against your natural instinct.

I really wanted to visit this particular place because it represented to me where it all started thousands of years ago—the human urge to face your fears in order to reach a different level of consciousness, which in my head equaled a life of bliss and freedom. It was the kind of life I wanted to live.

After a little convincing, I got the Bedouin guarding the entrance to remove the grid to the holy crocodile shaft. I could feel how my adrenaline was pumping. I wasn't expecting the shaft to be locked like this, and I didn't know for how long it had been closed off. I didn't know what was hiding down there. I could feel the fear in my body, and my brain was trying to tell me not to go down there. I was thinking, "Are there any spiders or scorpions down there? or snakes?"

There was no turning back now. I had come here to find it, and I was standing right in front of it. I took a deep breath through my nose and hurried down the hole. I had to crawl on my knees and elbows to move forward like a soldier in a trench. There was no water or crocodiles anymore, only darkness and desert sand. I could see the light in the other end about six meters ahead of me. I imagined how the initiate must have felt right before jumping into this hole for the first time not knowing what to expect and having to find the right way, while holding their breath.

The Fear Bucket List

I let go of my breath at the end like the initiate would have done. I did this as a symbol of my own initiation into my personal fear journey. This little experience of following in the Egyptian's footsteps, helped me to channel the energy I needed to proceed in my quest of facing my other fears. I felt like it was important to start my journey here, like so many before me thousands of years ago.

My fear of creepy crawlies had diminished, and it was replaced with happiness to be right there at that moment in this magnificent place.

With a quick *Sjukran* (thank you) to the Bedouin, I hurried back, while the desert sun set on the horizon. My ship was waiting, and I was the last one to return.

Chapter 8:
Mexico

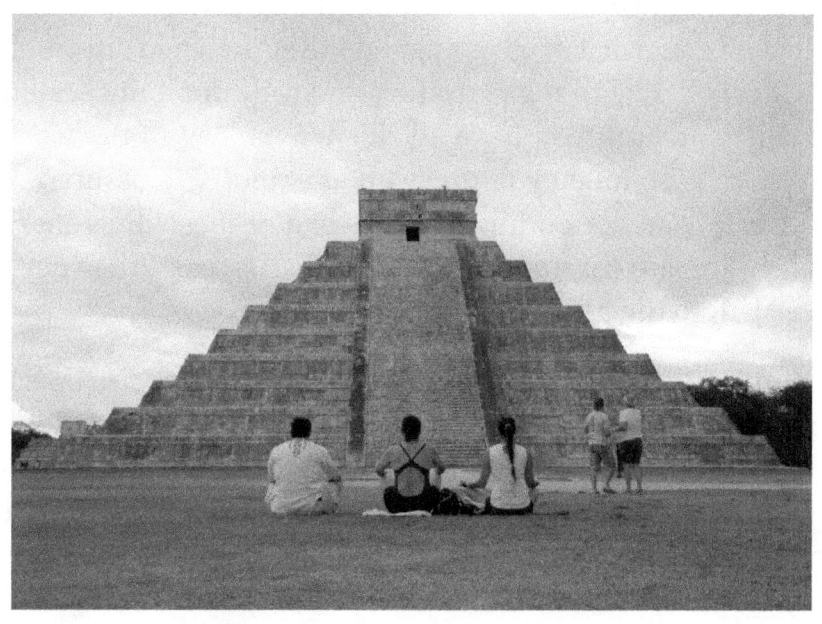

Castillo Pyramid - Chichen Itza

A couple of months before my Egypt journey, I was lucky enough to visit the indigenous Mayan people in Yucatan, Mexico.

This was a very special time for the Mayans because December 21st, 2012, was when their ancestor's calendar ended and a new cycle began.

If you remember, there were a lot of stories in the news about the end of the world and catastrophe movies in the cinemas creating fear. I decided to go to the source and find out what the fuss was about.

Chakras

When I first arrived in Mexico and had a chance to ask the elders about what was going on, they laughed and said, "Westerners like to make drama, and they don't understand what is going on. You have all this technology in the world, but there is so much you don't understand!" He assured me the world was not ending, but the age of masculine energy was ending after more than five thousand years, in order to give birth to the new feminine energy cycle.

The indigenous people of South America have a very special bond with nature and their ancestors. They live a simple non-materialistic life and have many different rituals that include the Earth and the sky. They call the Earth "Mother Earth" and the sky "Father Sky." They possess so much ancient knowledge that has been passed down from generation to generation.

The early Mayan religion mirrored the ancient Hindu; in fact, they might even predate it. Some believe the Mayans brought their culture to India. They talked about an

Chapter 8: Mexico

energetic anatomy of seven forces or energy centers in our body called the *Chacla* similar to the Hindu word *Chakra*.[16]

Chakra means spinning wheel in Sanskrit and refers to specific energy centers in the body. Each center is associated with a hormone gland in the endocrine system[17] in the body and corresponds to the spine. For example, the root chakra corresponds to the base of the spine, the pelvic floor, and the first three vertebrae. The chakras control the pranic energy within the body. Prana is seen as a universal energy considered as a life-giving force.

---

[16] *www.esotericonline.net*

[17] *The endocrine system is a collection of glands within the body that secrete more than twenty different hormones, known as chemical messengers, into the bloodstream.*

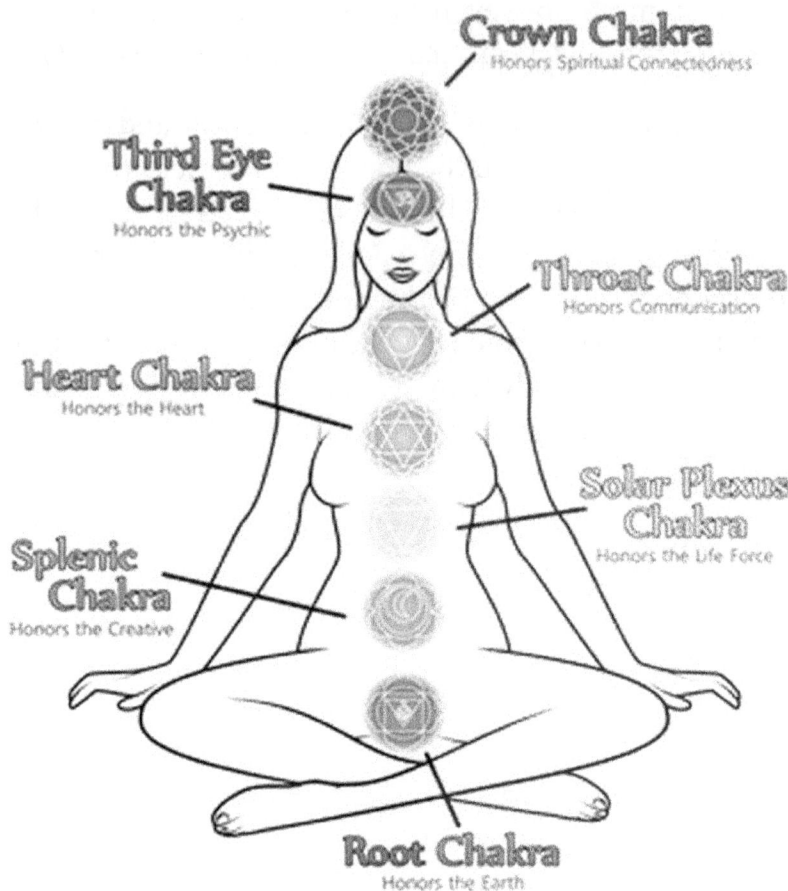

Crown chakra: pineal gland

Third eye chakra: pituitary gland

Throat chakra: thyroid/parathyroids

Heart chakra: thymus

Solar plexus chakra: pancreas

Splenic chakra: ovaries/testes

Root or base chakra: adrenals

When our chakras are in balance, so should the endocrine system be and vice versa. However, modern lifestyles are working against the equilibrium of our endocrine glands with things like BPA[18] from plastic bottles, pesticides in our food, and pollution in the air, which in turn will create a blockage and imbalance in our chakras.

For those who study the practice of yoga and/or meditation, it will come as no surprise that ancient yogis knew the chakras and endocrine system were interrelated and balancing the chakras was an integral part of a curative process for the endocrine system and thus for the whole body.

The chakras keep your body intact, as we know it. They all work at the same time but, as we grow up, they teach us different things in a natural order from the first chakra and upwards.

First Chakra: ROOT

This goes from your tailbone/base of the spine down your legs to your feet. This chakra roots you to the Earth like a tree roots itself to Mother Earth. The color is red like the core of the earth. To be rooted grounds you. This chakra has to do with FEAR, fight or flight, tribe, relationship with family. It is ruled by the adrenals/kidneys.

---

[18] *BPA: Bisphenol A – an organic synthetic compound/industrial chemical used in plastic bottles suspected to cause adverse health effects on the brain. www.mayoclinic.org*

Second Chakra: SPLEEN/PELVIC area

This one has to do with our emotions, intimacy, reproduction, creativity, money, and sexuality. This is where we create pleasure, children, songs, and business ideas. The color is orange. It is ruled by the ovaries/testes.

Third Chakra: SOLAR PLEXUS

This chakra has to do with ego, personal power, courage, fortitude, how you relate to yourself, and "having guts." It honors the life force. The third chakra allows you to meet challenges and move forward in your life. The color is yellow. This chakra is ruled by the pancreas.

Fourth Chakra: HEART

This one is unconditional love, primarily for yourself, your ability to protect yourself, and the capacity of non-judgment of your emotions. It is connected to loving yourself and others. You need to allow yourself to feel anger, sadness, happiness, and bliss. When you allow yourself to feel the feelings, you have self-acceptance. Then and only then can you live a life of loving kindness and compassion towards others. The color is green. It is ruled by the heart and thymus gland.

Fifth Chakra: THROAT

This one has to do with expression—the communication of our intention out into the world, being authentic, speaking the truth, and saying no when you need to. The main challenge in this chakra is doubt and negative thinking. The color is blue. It is ruled by the thyroid gland.

Chapter 8: Mexico

Sixth Chakra: THIRD EYE

This one represents intelligence. This is where you make decisions from and plan. It honors the psyche, the gift of seeing both inner and outer worlds. This is where you access inner guidance. The color is indigo. This chakra regulates all the hormones in your body, and it is ruled by the pituitary gland.

Seventh Chakra: CROWN

This one has to do with connecting to the source, an infinite spirit, experiences of unity, and a realization that everything is connected. This chakra is filled with serenity, peace, and joy. The color is violet (or sometimes white). It is ruled by the pineal gland that works as an inhibitor in the way that it controls the pituitary gland and inhibits the immediate discharging of thoughts into action and forces us to look inward in order to expand our consciousness.

Levels of foundational learning

First, at the root chakra you are building your foundation and then, as you branch out from your family, you are able to partner with the world (second). Then, you need courage to stand on your own two feet (third), stand up for yourself, and have good contact so people don't take advantage of you. Then, at the heart level (fourth), you pursue your joy, your bliss. It's about you, not what others want for you. Then, at the throat level (fifth), you speak your voice through your paintings, your films, and your business.

Then, at the third eye level (sixth), it's your capacity to envision the future, plan for it, and make it happen. It is psychic ability. The crown chakra (seventh) connects us to the infinite grid of possibility. Here we vibrate, we channel, and we receive inspiration and ideas. We bring in spirit expressed through our body.

We are energetic light beings, a system made of light. The opposite of light is the void. What makes you and I appear separate is that we have a different consciousness that allows us to come into physical form. But, if we look at you under a quantum physics microscope, you will see that you are nothing but vibrating particles of light.

Chakras are an *internal framework that the spirit hangs onto.*

When you understand that you have these levels of progression, you don't want to stay in the origin of your childhood, being a victim, or looking for mummy and daddy's approval at age fifty. You need to graduate, which means making money in the world, doing business with people, loving yourself, having a backbone, having an opinion, having an identity, and yet are not run by your ego.

We all need the ego to keep us alive. When running from a tiger, the ego is there to help, there in service to your unique identity. Yet, our work is to transcend the ego-based needs to **understand that we are infinite beings of light there to be in service to the unfolding of the infinite consciousness**.

Chakras can hold on to old *trauma and fear*. This can show itself as pain and tension in the body.

Chapter 8: Mexico

The next time you have a pain, notice where it is in the body and what chakra it is close to and try to see what the message is. You can become your own doctor like this by becoming aware of your own body and the signals it is giving you.

For example, if you break bones easily, this has to do with the seventh chakra/CROWN chakra. If left unattended, it can lead to depression and other mental disorders, and it can be triggered by a loss of purpose, an identity crisis, a lack of acceptance, being judgmental, or not caring for other people. Look into your connection to the Source or infinite spirit and ask yourself "Have I been acting selfish? Am I feeling let down/unsatisfied? Am I having trouble knowing what to do with myself?"

Imbalance of the Sixth chakra/THIRD EYE will manifest symptoms like tension headaches, migraine, visual defects, and sinus problems. It can be brought on by not trusting yourself or others, a lack of focus, a lack of direction, or a distraction. Look at trusting your intuition more and ask yourself if there is something else you would rather be doing.

Pain in the fifth chakra/THROAT occurs when you are having trouble expressing yourself or being unable to say what you want to say to others. It can appear as a tingling feeling, an unexpected cough, trouble swallowing, or feeling choked up. This can lead to thyroid problems (over active/under active), asthma, bronchitis, mouth ulcers, and sore throats.

89

Fourth chakra/HEART imbalance can show up as heart disease; allergies; cancer of the breast, lungs, or blood; and diseases of the immune system. It is usually caused by mistrust, lack of acceptance, bitterness, conditional love, and an emotional hurt. It is not a joke that you can die of a broken heart.

Stomach and intestinal problems, food allergies, diabetes, liver disease, and ulcers have to do with the third chakra/SOLAR PLEXUS. The imbalance is caused by low self-worth, worry about how other people view us, FEAR, and worry about the future. Look into your level of courage and fortitude. You must "have guts."

Symptoms like chronic lumbar spine pain, pre-menstrual syndrome, ovarian cysts, irritable bowel syndrome, and endometriosis can be linked to the second chakra/PELVIC area. Imbalances are usually caused by restrictions, low self-esteem, denial of pleasure, dependency, or issues with give and take. It can also mean problems with money.

Imbalance of the first chakra/ROOT or BASE chakra can manifest as problems in your hips, legs, knees, ankles, and feet. If not attended to, it can lead to constipation, Chrohn's disease, high blood pressure, impotence, weight issues, sciatica, addictions, and more. It is usually caused by a lack of safety, being worried, self-pity, doubting yourself, FEAR, or feeling low/depression. You should also look to see if there are any parts of your body you dislike, because this can also create an imbalance.

The indigenous people also taught me we are like an instrument; therefore, it is possible to heal a body with a specific vibration or sound. There are many great free sound healings on YouTube, all you need to do is search for it. I can really recommend listening to healing sounds on a regular basis.

I attended sacred ceremonies in the great Mayan temples with Mayan elder Don Pedro Pablo Chuc and a crystal skull ceremony with Hunbatz Men.

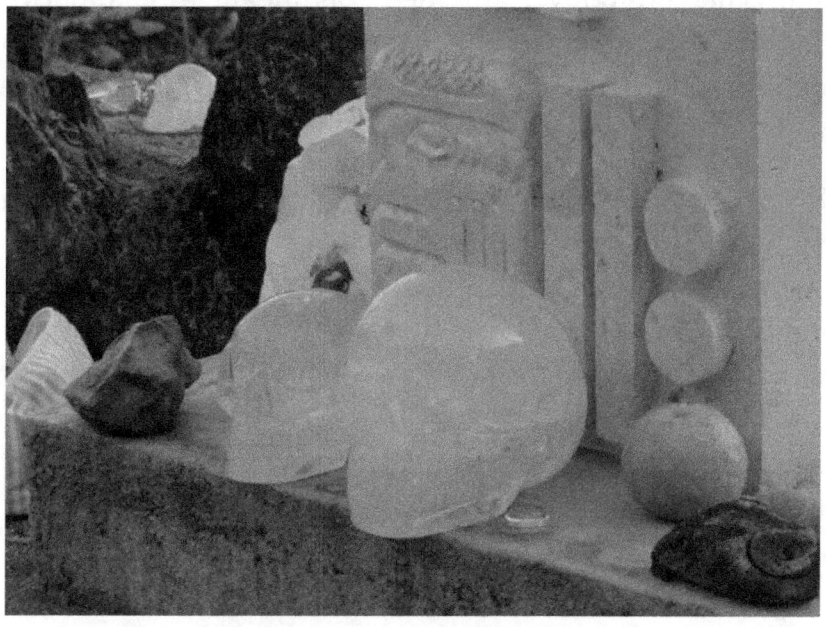

Ancient crystal skull ceremony

Crystal skull ceremony

During the visit in Yucatan, I participated in a sacred crystal skull ceremony. Allegedly, one of the original Mayan crystal skulls had been found in a private collection in France and returned to the elders. Many of the skulls have been lost or stolen and scattered around the world in the last centuries, but a few of them still remain.

No one knows for sure who made these skulls or when. The Mayans believed that there would come a time when thirteen crystal skulls would be reunited and change the world in the form of reawakening humanity. They believed the skulls contained vital information stored in the crystal itself. The ceremony I attended was meant to channel the energy of the remaining original skulls and welcome the new Feminine Cycle. It felt almost like being in an Indiana Jones movie.

To the nerds out there like me who are interested in learning the methods of the indigenous people, I suggest you look up a course on "awakening the illuminated heart" and go with a guide to these sacred places in Mexico. They have several trips every year. I can really recommend you to check out www.maureenstgermain.com for sacred journeys around the world. Maureen is really awesome and knows her stuff.

I travelled around Mexico and visited the many different temples all representing a different chakra.

In ancient times, the initiates would take this journey starting with the temple representing the base chakra and work their way up to the crown chakra temple. Like them, I went to all the temples and meditated in nature, to get in touch with my heart and the ancestors.

I really recommend taking this journey if you find yourself disconnected to your heart, like I was. It was definitely a heart opening experience, and I got in touch with myself in a

Chapter 8: Mexico

deeper way, which ultimately helped me conquer my fears. It is not a must to do this, but I felt a calling to go to these sites in order to get to the next level of my spiritual development.

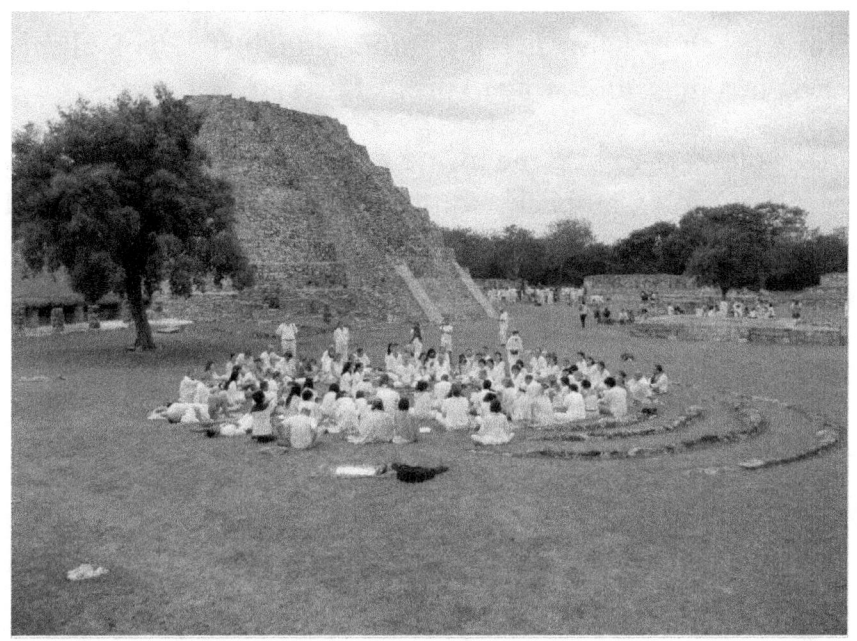

Mayapan

To finish the journey, we met with people from around the world on December 21st, 2012, at this temple site, where we did a huge beautiful meditation ceremony together.

It was a great sight with a giant circle of people, all dressed in white, from different nationalities coming together to welcome the new feminine cycle. Japanese women were dancing and playing the flute. Everyone was filled with unconditional love for each other and Mother Earth and Father Sky.

The Fear Bucket List

I'll never forget it. The energy and presence of the ancestors were a very special experience, and the ceremony helped me to get in touch with all the parts of my heart I had shut off years before. It helped me open my heart more instead of having a cage around it, and it also helped me become more aware of embracing my feminine side instead of always acting in a masculine way to protect myself.

Once you start to become aware of the love that we all truly are, there's no way back. You can't unlearn that or erase it from your memory.

Chapter 9:
Spirituality 101

"Once the soul awakens, the search begins and you can never go back."

John O'Donohue

I work as chiropractor in Hong Kong. Having a very Western medical and scientific background, but living in Asia where they focus more on holistic treatments, it is the perfect location for me, because it creates balance.

What most of my chiropractic colleagues back in Denmark don't know is that I also have a background in the spiritual world—a world I have already shared with you in the previous chapters about my travels.

I would like to share it even further with you, whether you are new to the spiritual world or experienced, or you can just skip this chapter and move on to the next one. It is completely up to you.

I believe the spiritual and physical world go hand in hand and one does not exclude the other. I think it's good to have a leg in both worlds in order to keep myself grounded, and I think the Eastern teachings and the Western teachings complement each other very well.

"We are not human beings having a spiritual experience but spiritual beings having a human experience."

Pierre Teilhard de Chardi (French philosopher)

Some people call it spirit, some call it soul, but it is the same. I will use the term spirit from now on, because I prefer this terminology.

Your spirit: the part of you that is eternal, immortal, and infinite. It is the part that accepts without judgment and loves without restriction.

The spirit is so powerful in energy that it would explode a physical body; therefore, it splits up into a reduced part of itself to take the human experience.

The spirit is the **REAL YOU**; it will always remain when everything else is gone.

Our desires come from our spirit. Nothing can exist outside of our spirit.

Our spirit communicates with us through intuition and feelings.

Higher self: the connecting link when the spirit speaks to the personality. The personality/spirit communication is the higher self-experience.

Chapter 9: Spirituality 101

Your higher self is that aspect of your spirit that is in you (when it split), but it is not the whole of your spirit.

The higher self is a part of you that is directly connected to the God force.

The difference between higher self and lower self can be described as follows:

Think of a nice road trip on the narrow and windy roads in the countryside. The radio is playing your favorite song, the sun is shining ... when, suddenly, you get a feeling you should slow down ... moments later a car comes towards you from the opposite direction with great speed swerving into your lane ... luckily, nothing happened because you had time to slow down and avoid the speeding car. This is lower self-communication.

Same scenario—you are driving down a country road when you're told to pull over and park, to stretch your legs, and enjoy the flowers in the fields. You do exactly that and the speeding car never gets in your way. This is higher self-communication. Higher self is able to see further ahead than lower self.[19]

Lower Self: is that sensory system that works outside of your five senses—the gut feeling or your intuition. Intuition serves your *survival*. It gives you hunches about danger ahead. The lower self keeps you safe, helps you understand life, and gives you information about physical safety or your

---

[19] Description of higher self from Maureen Saint Germain teleclass. See www.maureenstgermain.com for more details.

emotional body. It's a mix of your ego, physical, emotional, mental, and etheric body.

The Hawaiians describe the lower self as "the little girl/boy in you." Intuition is like a walkie-talkie between the personality and the spirit. This happens through the *higher self*.

The Ego: lives in the future and/or the past. It hates action, but likes living in the fantasy of doing it, talking about taking action but not doing anything about it. The ego is fear driven and compulsive and resides in the mental body.

The ego was created to design the illusion of separateness.

Your Personality: is the part of you that you were born into, that you live within and that will die in time. It is the vehicle of your evolution.

For each new incarnation/new life, the spirit creates a new personality in order to evolve and heal parts of itself.

After an incarnation, the spirit returns to its immortal state of love, compassion, and clarity.

Chapter 9: Spirituality 101

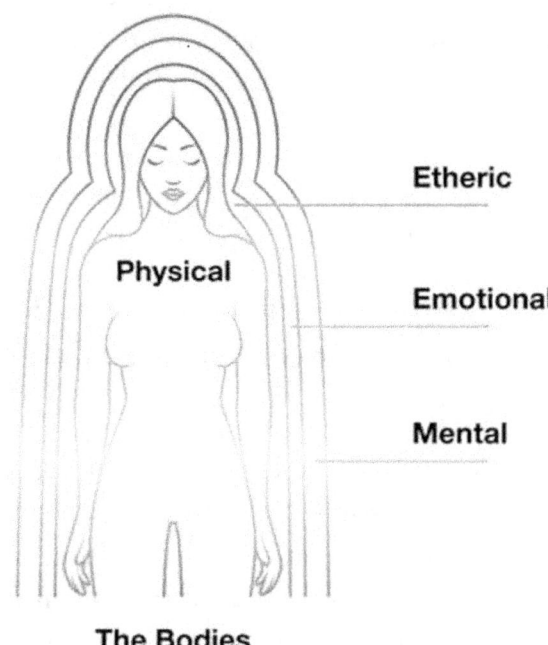

The Bodies

We have more than just one body; we have several layers just like an onion.

The Physical Body: what you can touch and feel, your arms, legs, torso and head, skeleton, muscles, organs, and skin.

The Etheric Body: our energy body, the part not yet in manifested form. It is your first link to your higher self and is comprised of energy that is in touch with all that is. The etheric body has centers of awareness and energy known as chakras.

The Emotional Body: our astral body. It represents the past. It stores feelings of past occurrences. Emotion is energy in motion that is qualified with a memory. Emotions must be felt to be cleared! Emotional healing is essential because your emotional wounds will keep you tied to the past.

To balance the emotional body, you need to start feeling good about yourself and forgive yourself.

The Mental Body: your mind or the vehicle of thought vibrations. This is where your thoughts of the past, present, and future linger.

How much power you have is correlated to the time it takes from thinking about something until it appears in your life, or is materialized. We call this timeline of thought to materialization *the metaphysical bank account*. If you have wasted energy in the past or waste energy in the future, you will have less metaphysical power.

"Reincarnation is the process that allows for the embodiment of the human soul for the purposes of self-realization."

Sufian Chaudhary

Frequency: you are a system of light! The frequency of your light depends on your consciousness. If you choose to feel forgiving, compassionate, joyful, or loving, you raise your frequency. If you choose feelings like hatred, jealousy, or **fear**, you lower your frequency, and emotional or physical disease will follow you.

Guides: each human has guides. A guide is an expert in an area that can be called in for consultation. For example, if you're writing a book or doing any other kind of project, you can call in a guide to give you creativity and insight. I regularly check in with my guides if I need direction during meditation.

Teacher: brings you closer to your spirit. The teacher brings you to the path of awareness and clarity. But remember, it is always you who makes the choice, not the guides or the teachers, as we are in a free-will zone here on Earth. Every decision you make either moves you towards your personality or towards your spirit.

Awakening: What is awakening? Awakening is a state of being of *remembering who you really are.*

It is not the role you "play" in this reality, such as mother, father, daughter, or son, and it is not your title either, such as I am a lawyer, I am a nurse, and so on. It is a pure being of who you are, that we are all equal by our birthright, and you are loved unconditionally, protected, secured, provided for, nurtured, and taken care of and that you are god-like, brilliant, magnificent, infinite, spiritual, physical, and a vibrational being.

You create this illusion of suffering on Earth in order to be aware of what you already are—*infinite love!*

Awakening is the key, a doorway toward higher consciousness and complete freedom from suffering, pain, and lack of the third dimensional reality, where most people live right now.

The Fear Bucket List

Many have already awakened and are seeking inward within the depths of their being to seek the solutions of their challenges in life.

There are many doorways that allow us to become awakened. By choosing to read this book, you are already on the path to awakening.

Chapter 10: Meditation

"The greatest power is surrender ..."

Deepak Chopra

Meditation has become very popular in recent years and is helping many people around the globe. It can offer significant benefits, from disease and pain management to better sleep, improved control of emotions, and even stress relief. It can sound like a wonder drug, but it might also sound like an impossible task when you can't—or don't have the opportunity to—sit still.

Some people make it sound so easy, to just sit down and meditate and clear out the mind of all your thoughts, but in reality, this can take some time to learn. It's like training your muscles in the gym. It takes practice, patience, and dedication, which most of us are not born with.

First encounter with meditation

One of the greatest gifts I have ever received was learning how to meditate!

I was twenty-three when I was introduced to a meditation teacher after someone close to me had tried to commit suicide. I didn't know how to deal with all the emotions and blamed myself for not being there to support her better.

My best friend was dating a guy who had a meditation group and suggested we go together and try it out. At first, I was reluctant, because I didn't like the idea of sitting in a group with my eyes closed, but I went anyway because I didn't want to disappoint my friend.

In the beginning, it was just a small group of six people meeting once a week and, because it was mostly the same people attending, I got to know them better and that made it easier for me to show up. Also, instead of just meditating, everyone got a chance to tell the group what their intention was for the day before the meditation. It was an invitation to tell the group what was going on inside and for many sessions I just listened to all the other group members talking about breakups, alcohol abuse, parent problems, etc. Every time I just chose to say, "My intention is to be right here, right now," which was basically a free pass if you didn't feel like sharing.

I had a million thoughts going through my brain. I was worried what the other people might think about me and kept thinking they were so much better at meditating than I was. They were older and more experienced. I just couldn't relax. Needless to say, this didn't help my meditation progress.

Fortunately, I was also stubborn, so I kept going to the weekly meditation group. Sometimes, I would fall asleep, sometimes my body would ache, sometimes I would relive being raped at age seventeen, and I would come out of the

Chapter 10: Meditation

meditation crying my eyes out. Sometimes, I would be six years old again and see my cousin in front of me.

One night something happened during the meditation practice, and I noticed a blissful feeling all over my body. That evening, I didn't want to come out of my meditative state when the teacher called us back to reality. That's when I realized that I had been meditating effectively and that meditation was actually pretty amazing.

Finally, one day I decided to share some of my story, and I remember how the teacher looked me straight in the eyes and said, "We attract exactly what we need in this life. You chose this before you even came into this life for yourself."

I felt like hitting him, the anger inside of me flared up and he could tell I was furious. How could anything that happened to me at such a young age, be something I attracted? I didn't understand so I just reacted, like I always did.

What he was trying to teach me was not to blame others for my misfortune and history, but to take responsibility one way or the other in order to start the healing process.

Later on, I contemplated the notion of choosing this incident as part of a bigger plan, and I decided in my mind that I was going to use it to help others.

Meditation has helped me overcome my fears by increasing my self-awareness and by guiding me to the next step, so I'm better prepared to take on the world. I have used meditation as my inner self-healing sanctuary, because it is always there, no matter what is going on around me. Every time I feel out of balance, I now notice it is usually after I have skipped my meditation practice for a few days. It is my body telling me to get back on track.

A regular meditation practice can have a whole host of benefits, but how do you manage to clear your mind in this million-miles-an-hour world with mobile phones giving you direct access to social media and tons of emails ticking in? Many people (including myself) have difficulty taking the time to tune out, because there are too many distractions. That is why I make a habit of scheduling my meditations, and I keep it down to maximum of twenty minutes a day. That way it doesn't feel overwhelming to me.

If you can't take twenty minutes for yourself, you don't have a life.

I don't care if you have to go sit on the toilet at work for twenty minutes to do your meditation, just get it done, and you will see how this habit can change your life.

I have meditated for ten years now and am acutely aware of the power of meditation. I find it clears my mind and makes me more present in the now. It balances out the inevitable stress in my everyday life and gives me better coping skills when something unexpected comes up. This experience made me believe that you should always practice what you are not good at, instead of always doing what you know. This is an important step in our journey here on Earth, just like love and compassion and facing your fears. And, seriously, if I could learn to meditate, so can YOU! I promise!

Chapter 10: Meditation

So if you want to start your meditation journey, here are my pointers for getting started:

How do I meditate?

First of all, forget about sitting crossed-legged or in lotus position unless you are an experienced yogi or very flexible! There are many meditation traditions that tell you that you must sit in a certain way to experience enlightenment and the benefits of meditation, but I don't agree with this.

It's perfectly okay to sit on a normal chair in an upright position with your feet on the ground. But do try to sit upright, as this ensures the 'chi' (the life-giving energy that unites body, mind, and spirit) in your body to flow freely. It's quite important to have a balanced spine with no blockages. If you're out of alignment in your spine, your chi will be disrupted and you'll feel discomfort during meditation.

Try to avoid supporting your back with pillows, because in my experience, you'll find yourself snoring after five minutes if it's too comfortable. But it's very important not to be in pain either, as this will disrupt your meditation experience. Find a balance where you are comfortable, but not too comfortable.

In the beginning, it can be a little hard to start meditating in silence. I suggest you start out with some relaxing meditation music (you can find a great deal on YouTube) or even listen to a guided meditation.

Start with fifteen to twenty minutes and gradually increase your meditation time to whatever suits your life and schedule. I will usually do a daily twenty minutes meditation and then a longer one on the weekend or whenever time allows me to meditate longer.

Close your eyes and take some deep breaths to connect with your body. Feel your body. Is there any tension or discomfort? Notice what's going on as you move your focus up and down your body, like a CAT scan done by yourself.

Focus on your breath, breathing in and out of your nose. Feel the sensation in your nostrils when the air enters and leaves again. Accept that there can be noise around you, but preferably meditate in a quiet environment without disturbances in the beginning.

Be present in the moment. Commit to being right here, right now for the time you have agreed—it doesn't matter if it's fifteen minutes or two hours. Turn your phone to silent mode, not vibration. Know that it's okay to fall asleep, fall off the chair, be bored, cry, have thoughts, worry about your grocery shopping, etc. It's completely normal in the beginning and sometimes later on as well—we're still human, after all.

When you have a thought, acknowledge that thought and let it go, let it drift away like clouds in the sky. If you keep thinking "I must clear my mind and think of nothing," guess what? You'll have a stream of thoughts coming your way, so just relax and let them slowly float away.

Find a meditation place that suits you, whether it is a special place in your apartment, in your office with a closed door (toilet), or on the beach somewhere. I often travel to different places in order to immerse myself in meditation in nature. Nature has the ability to really ground you and fill you up with energy.

Try meditating in a group. It's easier to keep up the energy in a group because everyone is helping each other. It's like pushing a car up a hill. It's very hard to do alone. A group of people will find it much easier.

Know that you are not here to gain anything specific. Trying to accomplish a certain state or feeling will screw up your meditation because you will be all in your head ... but it's okay if it happens. Be gentle on yourself and learn from it.

Benefits of meditation

- Better sleep
- Sharper decision making
- Improved concentration
- Greater productivity
- More control of emotions
- Stress relief
- Connection with yourself
- Improved ability to be present in the moment
- Takes us beyond our worries, fears, and judgments
- Better knowledge of our inner self/awakening
- Increased production of anti-aging hormone DHEA
- Disease and pain management—self-healing
- Alters the structure of the brain to the better

The Fear Bucket List

So, no more excuses. Just do it! Go on, I believe in you! Start your meditation journey today. You will get addicted to this time for yourself and the benefits it will give you.

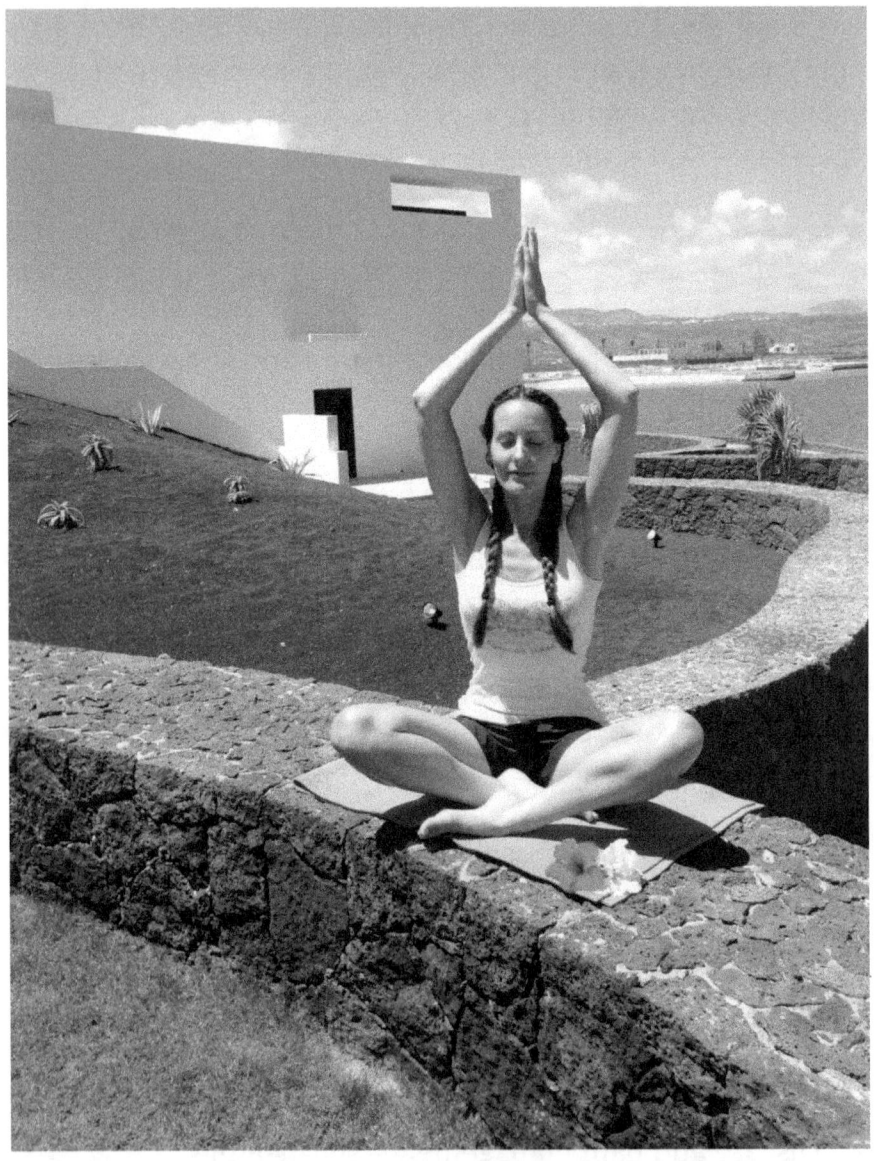

Meditating

Chapter 10: Meditation

Connecting with your spirit requires you to create some space for allowing you to focus on yourself. Meditation is a proven technique that helps clear your mind, focus on your life, and clarify where you wish to go.

Meditation will create an inner contact and teach you to master your emotions.

Meditation can help you accept your reality and let go of the energy caused by negative thoughts and emotions stored in your physical body like fear or hurt.

Meditation lowers brainwave frequency, gives you inner peace, excess energy, and insight into what really matters in your life.

Meditation is a great way to maintain your center and balance in your life and can have great prophylactic effect on your body preventing diseases.

The question is: will you choose the way of doubt and fear or will you choose the path of wisdom? This is a free-will zone, meaning it is really up to you to make the decision. If you need help, ask your guides and teachers for help.

Fear is a gateway to a higher self-awareness. So, in a way, it's a good thing. You can use it to your advantage by acknowledging the fear when it comes up and facing it.

Facing your fear is a way to separate yourself from the mass consciousness, the *lemmings*.

As I said earlier, there are many doorways to reach awakening, such as losing someone close to you, being raped,

The Fear Bucket List

having a near-death experience, losing all your belongings, or going bankrupt. Trauma can create awakening by forcing you on a path of self-awareness, but let's try to do this through meditation first.

Meditation can really help you on your journey to self-healing and self-empowerment and, if you combine it with facing your fears, you will get there much faster. This has been my recipe of overcoming both child molestation, domestic violence and rape. It's like a **spiritual shortcut to awakening and bliss.**

But note that if you feel like you are not up to doing it all by yourself, please contact an organization like www.rainn.org for free online hotline help or a professional psychotherapist.

I have also created a guided Higher Self meditation for you. Go to www.thefearbucketlist.com to download it and use it in your own time.

Part IV – The Fear Bucket List

"Fear is not real. The only place that fear can exist is in our thoughts about the future. It is a product of our imagination causing us to fear things that do not at present exist and may not ever exist. That is near insanity. Danger is very real, but fear is a choice."

Will Smith in the movie *After Earth*.

If you really want to go from victim to power woman and set yourself free, you have to destroy your fears one way or the other! We have the meditation down; now it's time for some action!

As I told you in the beginning, there are many ways to lift your consciousness and empower yourself; this is just my recipe of a shortcut to the amazing world of higher consciousness and bliss, a life where fear isn't holding you back from a life of freedom.

My Fear Bucket List transformed my life by helping me overcome the larger fears in my life, and it is meant to be an inspiration to you. Every time I faced a fear on the list, I felt more and more empowered and all the things that happened to me in the past became more and more insignificant. It helped me step out of the victim role.

Everyone has their own individual fears, and I know there is a big difference between being afraid of heights and having social anxiety, so I strongly recommend that you create your own personalized Fear Bucket List to suit your needs best.

I know not everyone can afford travelling around the world. I couldn't, but I worked very hard and spent every single holiday I had on facing my fears. I even maxed out my credit cards (not recommended), but I did what I had to and invested in myself in order to make this happen, because it was important for me in order to live the life I knew I could have, without anything or anyone holding me back.

I still add things and experiences to my Fear Bucket List as I get older. It's a lifelong process. All you can do is your best.

I suggest you start by writing some things down that you are scared of, whether it is heights or walking into a crowded room. Then commit to facing them in our Facebook community (www.facebook.com/TheFearBucketList) or tell a close friend or family member, who can keep you accountable. Maybe you can even have someone join you on your adventures and you can face your fears together.

When I faced my fear of sharks, my friend joined me on the boat out there facing her own fear of falling in the water. She had fallen overboard once and was stuck in shark infested waters for hours before being rescued. We helped each other follow through and not chicken out.

Chapter 11:
Fear of White Sharks

"You gain strength, courage, and confidence by every experience in which you really stop to look fear in the face."

Eleanor Roosevelt

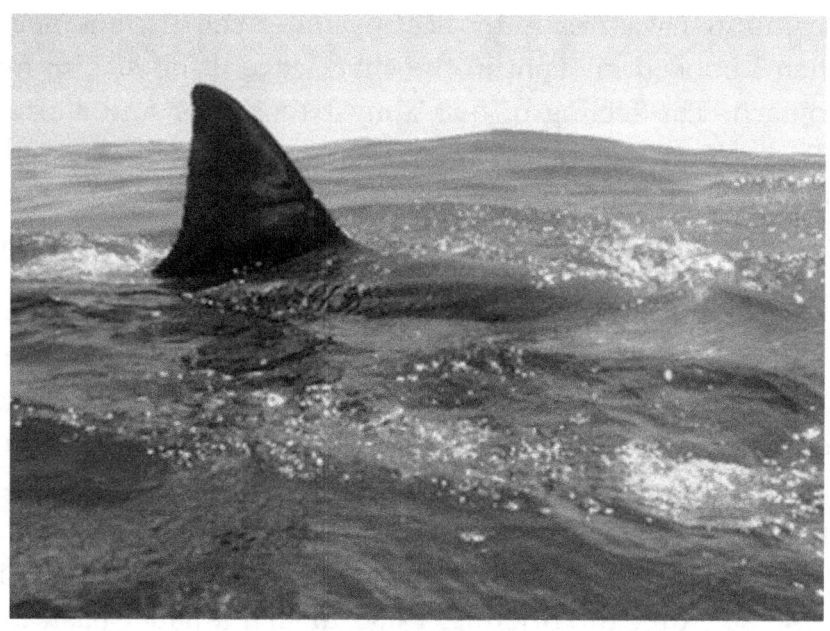

Female white shark circling the cage

The Fear Bucket List

One day I was watching an animal program on National Geographic channel showing a great white shark, filmed for the first time, coming up vertically from the deep and breaching the water. It jumped almost completely out of the water, from nose to tail, and grabbed a seal in its jaws, before it splashed down again making a huge wave. I jumped off the sofa, and I remembered thinking wow! that must be super scary to see in real life. It was something I would never do, but then I remembered my promise to myself about starting to face my fears and empower myself, and I started planning my trip with the purpose of overcoming my fears.

I started my Fear Bucket List journey in the beautiful country of South Africa, one of my favorite places on Earth. It took encountering one of the most feared animals face to face, until I was ready to face my inner self. I remember, when I booked my spot in the shark cage, I felt sick to my stomach. The feeling of fear almost took over and started talking to me saying, "Why are you doing this to yourself? You don't need to do this! What is wrong with you?" But I was determined to prove that I could do anything I wanted to!

I didn't sleep much the night before and, on the day of the cage diving, I got up really early and drove to Gainsbaai, South Africa, where some of the world's best cage diving takes place. We had a quick briefing before the dive, important things like don't try to feed the shark and stay in the cage; if you stick your hands out, the shark *will* bite it off or worse! After the briefing, I had to sign a paper basically saying, if I died out there, it was my own responsibility. As

Chapter 11: Fear of White Sharks

you can imagine, this didn't exactly settle my nerves. I could feel my stomach rumbling, and my head felt light. It was as if my body had a mind of its own.

We sailed out to Dyer Island also known as Seal Island. The waves were huge, and I was very pleased that I had taken a seasick tablet as a precaution earlier that morning. I immediately recognized the place from National Geographic. The spot was perfect, right between Dyer Island and Geyser Rock where a colony of 60,000 Cape Fur Seals breed. This place is known as Shark Alley.

There was another couple on the boat who were supposed to go in the water, but they were already very seasick and stayed on the boat. So, there I was, one Scandinavian girl with a huge cage in front of me.

I quickly put my wetsuit on and jumped in. I knew the crew had been putting blood and fish bait in the water to lure the sharks in but, at first, I couldn't see anything. The water was very cold and murky, but I knew there were sharks there. I knew, because I could feel the little hairs on my neck rising.

The cage was banging into the side of the ship because of the waves, and I had to hold on with all my power to keep my legs from popping out between the metal bars. I managed to get my legs under control and, just like that, out of nowhere, the great white came from the deep black water and went for the bait on the surface. It must have come from underneath, just as I had seen on TV. But this time I was right in front of it. I could almost touch it, and the impact of this giant shark, when it landed in the water, was so amazing!

The Fear Bucket List

I quickly forgot about my fear and started to enjoy the interaction with these intense great creatures and felt very grateful to experience their presence in their own environment. They were very curious and came right up to the cage to investigate. I had eye contact with a huge female and forgot to breathe in awe of how close she was to the cage. I could almost touch her. It was so incredible.

I could feel my heart beating, but I managed to stay calm until they dragged me up from the cage, because I was starting to get hypothermia from the cold water. I didn't want to miss a second of this, and I definitely learned that the great white looks much bigger in real life than on TV.

I congratulated my friend for facing her fear of boats and myself for being able to cross out the first major fear on my Fear Bucket List and moved on to planning my next adventure.

Chapter 12:
Fear of Small Spaces
(Cave Diving)

"The journey away from ego toward spirit is a journey through fog. You're only going to see a few steps in front of you."

Stuart Wilde

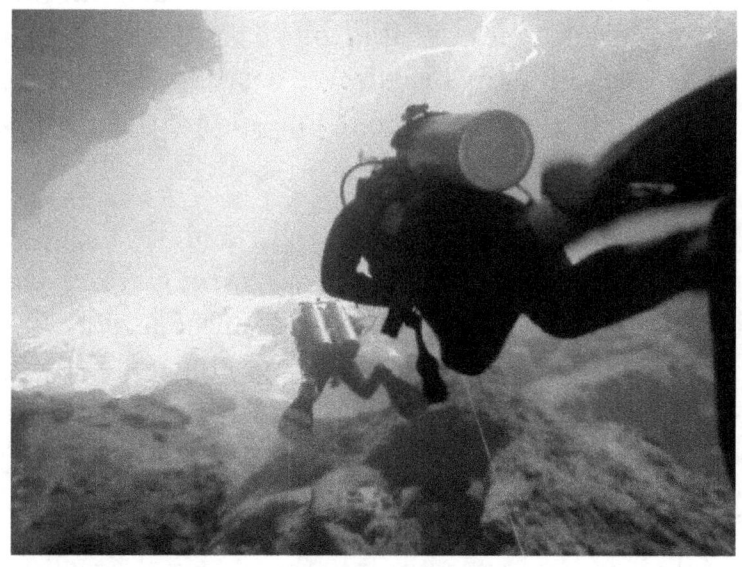

Cave diving

The Fear Bucket List

Since I was thirteen, I have dived in the ocean, but I wanted to try something new and scary. I had heard about cave diving, but never tried it. I had heard it was a very dangerous sport and people had died exploring the underwater caves. This made it a perfect Fear Bucket List adventure.

I booked my ticket and went to Yucatan in Mexico to face my fear of small spaces and darkness.

When I first met my cave dive instructor, I was surprised; she was a local woman, about 170 cm tall, with a small build, and a great smile on her face. Her name was Candy Lopez. I could tell she was doing something she absolutely loved, and she seemed very excited to show her caves to me.

We drove into the jungle and geared up in our wetsuits. We had to walk for a while to reach the cave, and then jump down two meters from the edge. It was challenging in the humidity and heat and, by the time I entered the water, I was already catching my breath. We descended about thirty-five meters all the way down to the bottom of this freshwater hole in the middle of the jungle.

During the last couple of meters, the visibility disappeared, and it looked like we were descending through thick clouds. The bottom was muddy and dark and, in the middle, a great tree was lying peacefully, it had probably fallen in there many years ago. It looked like a ghostly realm, and I decided to ascend to brighter waters.

Further up there was an entrance in the side of a vertical wall. I followed my instructor into the hole in the wall, and it

Chapter 12: Fear of Small Spaces

continued in like a pathway of tunnels until it led us out further up in the water hole.

It was amazing to swim in this dark hole, not knowing what was waiting for us.

The hard part was getting out of the hole by dragging myself up on a rope with my arm muscles, with all the diving equipment on my back, and hiking back to the car. Afterwards I felt thrilled to have done it, and I couldn't wait to see the next cave.

The next one was very different, and I had to stay close to the instructor as we moved further and further into the cave, this time there was no way up. There was only one way— following the little white string on the bottom of the cave. The string was there so that no diver would get lost in these giant caves with many pathways like a labyrinth. There were big warning signs telling us not to go into certain tunnels because of great danger.

Even swimming with the fins was different in these caves, because it was very important not to kick up the mud and make visibility low; instead, I had to kick like a frog. I noticed that, in some places, the water felt cold and, in other places, it was lukewarm. Sometimes there were beautiful rays of sunlight coming from holes above and sometimes it was pitch black, and I had to turn on my torch to see my instructor's air tank. It was super scary at first, but I felt like the more time I spent in the caves, the more relaxed my body became.

The Fear Bucket List

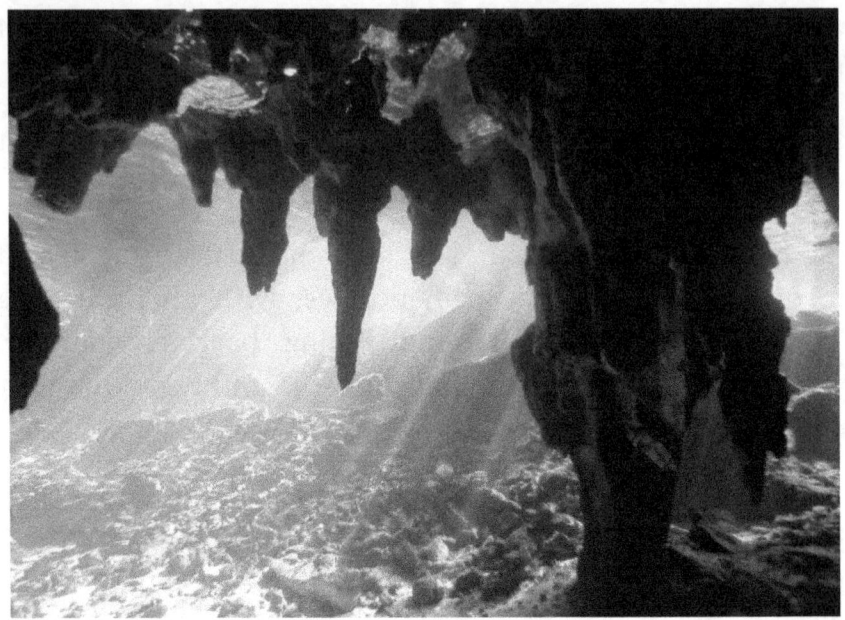

Rays of sunlight in Ponderosa Cavern, Yucatan

There is no room for panic in a cave, so you just keep moving forward and take it slow.

It was a great lesson for me to learn. I use this metaphor in my day-to-day life, when I feel like I need to be more patient in a situation or with certain people.

At a point in the dive, the water became blurred, like if you were wearing contacts and they suddenly fell out of your eyes. It was a very strange sensation, and I could feel my heart beating faster. Not knowing what it was, I just kept swimming until, all of a sudden, the water was crystal clear!

My instructor later told me that this phenomenon was called *halocline,* and it was where the fresh water and salt water

Chapter 12: Fear of Small Spaces

met. Haloclines are common in water-filled caves near the ocean. Less dense fresh water from the land forms a layer over salt water from the ocean. For underwater cave explorers, this can cause the optical illusion of air space in caverns. Passing through the halocline tends to stir up the layers.

After five days of exploring caves in Mexico, I no longer had any fear of small spaces or darkness—mission accomplished! It was another fear to cross off my Fear Bucket List.

Chapter 13:
Fear of Heights

"Whether you believe you can do a thing or not, you are right."

Henry Ford

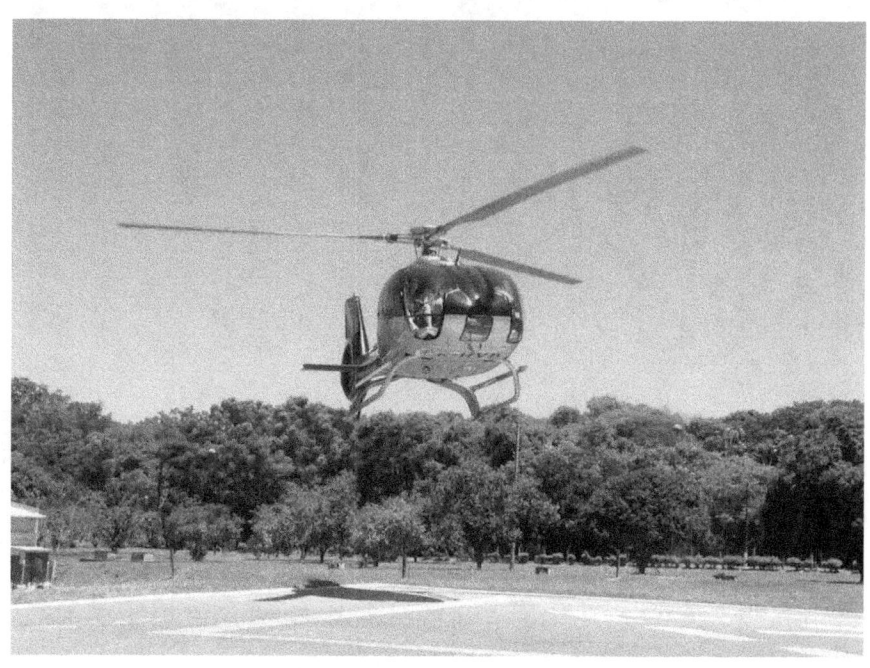

My helicopter ride

The Fear Bucket List

My trip to Argentina was amazing. I got to face my fear of heights in three different ways.

The first one was flying over the beautiful Iguazú waterfalls in a helicopter. I got to sit in front and had the best view but, being scared of heights, that was not necessarily a good thing! Even the bottom of the helicopter was Plexiglas, so it was a bit intimidating to sit there and look down. My brain kept thinking *What if we crash*? But the longer I sat there, the more I enjoyed it. It was a breathtaking view after all, and the pilot seemed very experienced.

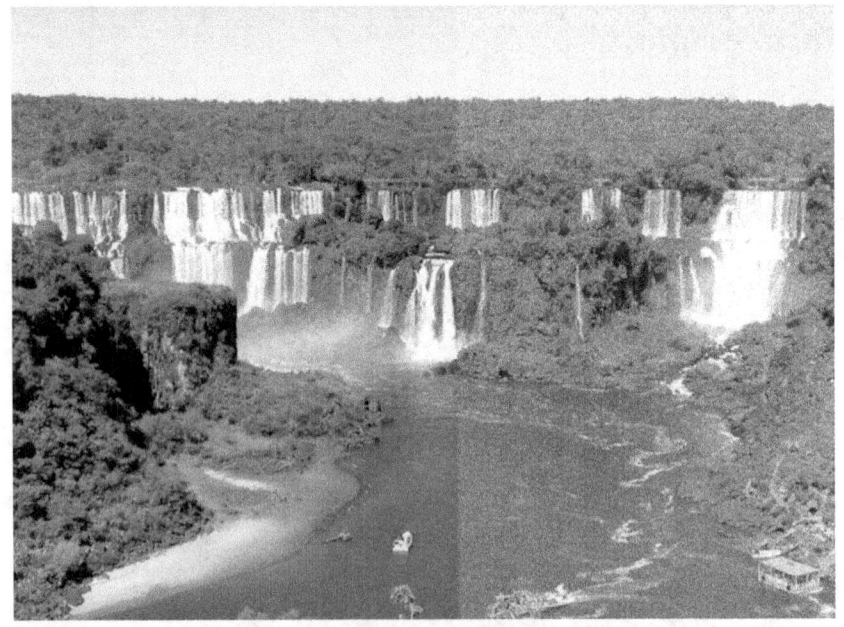

Iguazú waterfalls from above

After trekking around on the ground for hours seeing and feeling the power of the waterfalls, it was fantastic to go in

Chapter 13: Fear of Heights

the helicopter and experience it all from a different perspective. But it definitely made my stomach turn!

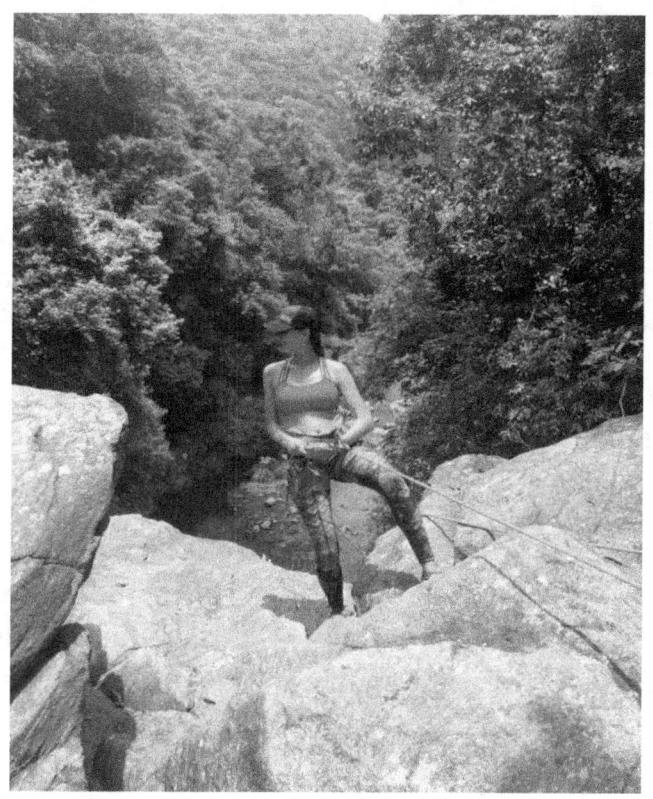

Canyoning

A couple of days later, I joined an adventure tour through the jungle, where we trekked to a waterfall. The idea was to rappel down the waterfall; some people call it canyoning. I really like water, but not heights, so I thought this would be a great way to challenge myself. Plus it was really hot and humid outside, so I didn't mind a little swim.

I was confident until we reached the waterfall. I didn't expect it to be so high up and the rocks seemed very slippery where the water had shaped them for many years. I sat down on a rock on top and gathered my courage.

I waited a little while, until I was the last one standing. I wanted to make sure the rope was okay.

Finally, I decided to go for it and turned my back to the falling water, pushed against the rocks with my feet, and descended. The water was really cold and had great power. I had to hold on tight to the rope, and I was concentrating so hard, I managed to forget my fear and actually enjoy it.

Before I knew it, I was all the way down, and I was sure my fear of heights was gone ... but there was only one way to test it.

The next day, I drove a Jeep into the jungle again, but this time it was time to try a cableway **high up under the trees. I guess it was hanging about twenty to thirty meters up in the air. The guide started by giving us our safety gear with a harness** and a helmet. Then he said, "If you go up the first stairs to the platform, there is no turning back, you have to continue on the track, there will be no exits until the last platform."

Great! No way back, I liked that! It was good when you wanted to push yourself.

I could feel my legs starting to shake when I climbed the narrow wooden ladder leading up to the first platform, so I guess there was still some fear left. On my left, giant jungle ants were walking side by side with me. They didn't seem bothered by the height at all.

Chapter 13: Fear of Heights

While standing on the platform, a guy attached me to the thick metal wire. I could see it went a long way into the green treetops, but I couldn't see the ending. Before I knew it, I was on my way, flying through the jungle attached to a wire with a single harness. I forgot to brake and almost knocked the guy off the next platform.

Each time I jumped off one platform to glide to the next, my fear changed again to excitement and a happy, free feeling inside. I was completely present in the now—like nothing else mattered. It was a great experience, and it cured the last bit of my fear of heights.

Chapter 14:
Fear of Crashing

"When a person really desires something, all the universe conspires to help that person to realize his dream."

Paulo Coelho

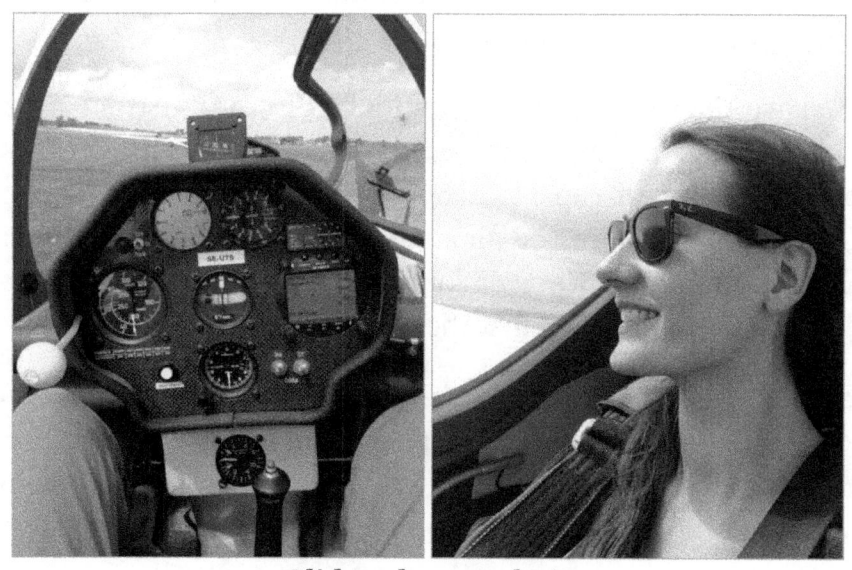

Glider plane cockpit

The Fear Bucket List

My fear of flying was tested a couple of months later, when I was invited to go in a glider plane. At first I was reluctant ... why would I go into a very small aircraft with no engine? It seemed a bit silly to test fate but, ever since I started this journey of crossing off everything on my Fear Bucket List, I've noticed that I agree to try more than I did before. It's like a calling and, on the positive side, I get to share it with you.

It was a beautiful summer day with only a few cumulus clouds in the sky. When I arrived at the glider plane club, people were already preparing the glider planes. Little red propeller planes took turns to drag the glider planes up in the air behind them. They were lining up on the runway, eager to get up there in the sky and fly like a bird.

I was strapped in tight in the plane. The pilot said it was to avoid hurting my head on the ceiling. I was wondering what he meant, but I found out later!

He gave the okay signal to the pilot in front of us flying the old propeller plane. It started moving fast and dragged us behind it with a rope attached to the front of our plane. Once we were up in the air high enough, my pilot let go of the rope, and we were on our own. There were no more engines keeping us up, just the different air streams.

Gliding is all about finding the thermals in order to stay up longer. If you don't find these pockets of rising air, the plane will drop in altitude, and you will be back on the ground in no time.

Chapter 14: Fear of Crashing

I understand why people are drawn to this sport; it is so quiet and beautiful up there. It's like a completely different world. Looking out of the glass ceiling, I could see big falcons playing in the thermals like us. When entering a big cloud, the plane would very quickly rise in altitude and give a rush to the stomach. It felt like a roller coaster ride.

I was really enjoying it but, all of a sudden, I was hanging upside down! The pilot had made a loop, and I understood why my seatbelt had to be so tight! I screamed out loud in shock. I could feel all my blood pooling in my head and started feeling a little nauseous. After a while, I got used to the feeling and enjoyed every loop and fall in altitude. He even let me steer the plane myself, which was awesome! When we landed safely on the ground, I was completely high on life from all the adrenalin pumping through my system.

* * *

I have always been scared of crashing in a car as well as in an airplane, so I decided to conquer this fear the following weekend by going to a racetrack in the Swedish countryside where all the guys went on the weekends to drive their sports cars around legally at full speed. I decided it would be fun to go try it out and got in contact with a professional racecar driver. He agreed to take me around the track in his Porsche, a car he had custom made with all these extra gadgets and more horsepower in order for it to be super powerful.

I strapped in and put my helmet on. Two seconds later, he pushed the gas pedal down to the max. I was moving around so fast in my seat to the right, then to the left, that I had to hold on to the door during the turns. It was like being in a computer game, but in real life with the same view as the player. The only difference was here, if you made a mistake, it would be game over for real.

I think I was screaming around half the track every time we hit a turn but, eventually, after a couple of laps, I trusted the driver and let go. It was so much fun and driving home in my own car seemed like such an anti-climax!

Chapter 15:
Fear of Being Alone

"People who have been through ultimate pain psychologically, sexually, spiritually, or emotionally often become the people who contribute the most to society ..."

Anthony Robbins

My worst break up was after two years of a really passionate relationship. My boyfriend and I had moved to Sweden together because he was finding it hard to get a job in Denmark. I paid for everything for a while, because he was between jobs at the time. But when we arrived in Sweden, he finally got a job, and we decided to start a chiropractic clinic together as partners. I let him handle the financial side of the business, so I could focus on healing my patients.

I was the one taking the loans at the bank to start the business up because I was already working full time for another company. He assured me that I would get it back once the business started earning money. I didn't mind. I was so in love it didn't matter. He helped out by contributing with his paychecks as well, so we could pay for a couple of employees in the clinic from the beginning.

The Fear Bucket List

I really believed it would be a success. And it was for almost a year. It was hard in the beginning, because I was running the clinic and still working part time in Denmark, plus taking care of his six-year-old daughter every other weekend, while he played computer games.

I had many new clients and thrived working in my own clinic.

We were best friends, had so much passion, and shared the need for exploring. We travelled together when we had the chance, and I really thought he cared for me, and it would last forever. But, one day when the business began to earn money, he started getting very controlling and violent and wanted to have full ownership in our mutual company.

I knew he still owed money for his boat and car, but I figured he had things under control. By that time, I had just quit my part-time job and focused one hundred percent on our clinic. So, when he said it would be better if he just owned the company and all I had to do was sign some papers, I was a bit confused. It just didn't make any sense to me.

I went from having the best time of my life, to one morning being woken up at 6 a.m. and thrown on the floor by him in our apartment. He literally lifted me up and threw me on the floor, and then he tried to force me to sign a paper that let him take over the company. I just couldn't believe he wasn't satisfied with owning fifty percent and, of course, I refused to sign the papers. His response was to try to force me again by using more violence including strangulation, and I ended up struggling with him on the floor until I got

Chapter 15: Fear of Being Alone

away and locked myself in the bathroom. I stayed there until I could hear he had left, and I felt safe to come out.

Needless to say, I left him the same day! Bruised and hurt, I packed whatever I could carry into the car and drove away from everything. I left immediately on a two-week vacation with my family, and he closed the company with a lawyer he was sleeping with, while I was away, so I had nothing to come back to. I should have known something was up, but I didn't. I was too tired and stressed to notice he was seeing other women behind my back and plotting how to get rid of me with a profit.

It took a lot of guts to make that decision, and I know many women before me would have chosen to stay and figure things out, like my grandmother had done for many years back in the day. She was beaten every day, by her ex-husband but still hoped that the father of her twins would come to his senses. Because I had trained myself to react in fearful situations, I took action and left, even though my heart was completely broken, and all I had left was a couple of things and a huge personal debt.

It was the lowest I had ever been, and ***I had to start over again from scratch! Everything I had built was taken away from me in an instant.*** I couldn't even contact my patients to tell them why the clinic was closed, as I didn't have access to the computers anymore—he made sure of that—and it really hurt me not being able to communicate with them.

It's funny how decisions about love hurt the most. It felt like my whole existence was threatened. All I could feel was a huge hole in my chest and a disappointment of what I had lost—love and my company (my precious company that I had built from the ground up). I was also scared to be alone. I was scared I wasn't good enough, and all those self-destructive thoughts came up after the break up.

But this is what I learned: life doesn't end, even though your relationship ends. It might feel like it in the moment, because you were used to the certainty of waking up next to someone. You might be scared to let go of your certainty and comfort zone, but it's worth it if you do dare to make the jump.

Many people, including myself at an earlier age, fall into the trap of staying in a relationship way too long, because the pain of making the decision to leave exceeds the pain of staying. So, we come up with excuses to stay even though, deep in our hearts, we know it's not working. So, we end up suffering, not being ourselves, and playing an act of being happy when we're not, instead of just taking action on the message we're being given.

Does it sound familiar? Maybe it does and maybe it doesn't. Maybe this has just been the case for me. But maybe you do recognize this pattern or know someone who is stuck in between. Maybe you can help by making them more aware, or maybe you can just support them and ease the transition when the decision has been made. It is really important to have good people and family around for support, even though, in the end, the transition is entirely up to you.

Sometimes losing it all gives you an opportunity to start fresh. Sometimes it's a present in disguise!

Chapter 16:
Fear of Not Being Good Enough

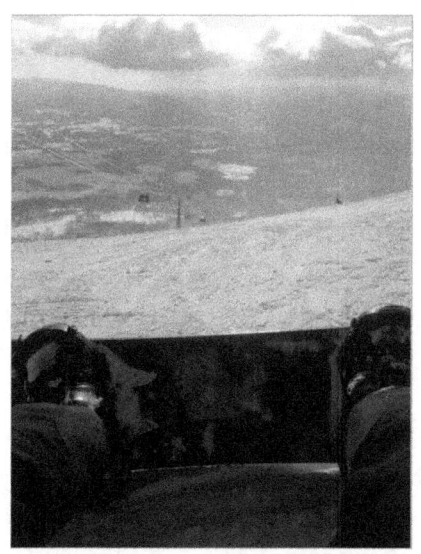 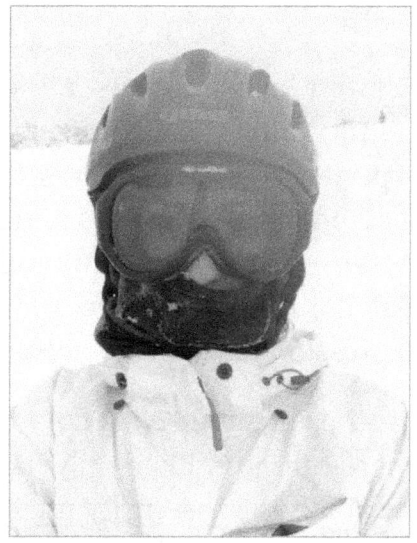

Ready for my first run in Niseko, Japan

After a while on my own, I met a fantastic man. Very early into the relationship he surprised me with an invitation to go to Japan for a week to snowboard and celebrate New Year's Eve. I had always wanted to see Japan, so I accepted the invitation with pleasure, and we arrived in beautiful

The Fear Bucket List

snow-white Sapporo, Japan, and drove a couple of hours to Niseko.

I was feeling a little excited and nervous inside at the same time. "What if I'm not good enough? What if I fall and break a leg?" It's that annoying little voice of fear I still get, when I'm trying something new (I call it "little-me"). I wonder if it will always be there, or if it will fade in time, as I pursue the remaining fears on my bucket list. Time will tell.

I went to the rental place and got my gear ready. I certainly looked the part, but *is this really a good idea?* I thought to myself.

Before I knew it, I was in the gondola on my way to the top of the mountain with my man and his friend, both experienced snowboarders. They were already talking about the off-piste snowboarding (snowboarding ungroomed terrain) on powder snow, and they seemed so fearless. I was jealous; I wanted to feel that way too, so I used their facial expression to motivate myself.

On top, it was very windy, and I was struggling to put my board on right, I had only had two hours of private tutoring, and I felt the insecurity creeping up, but I pushed it aside. I remember my father always said, "What can you do about it? Nothing! So, move on."

I continued for about ten meters, before I tumbled and fell hard. I decided to get up and not think too much about it and continued my journey down the mountain. I kept falling over when I turned—sometimes I edged my board and fell backwards, and sometimes I did a full circle with legs and

Chapter 16: Fear of Not Being Good Enough

board in the air. It felt a little like a metaphor for my life—falling over but always getting up again.

One fall was so hard my phone stopped working, and my shoulder took a beating. But, no matter how hard I fell, I got up again and continued. I refused to let the fear get the best of me. I would not give up! I knew that my balance and muscle memory would get better and better, and I was determined to have that same facial expression of happiness, like the guys in the gondola earlier.

Every single turn for the first two days made my adrenalin pump, because I didn't know if I would make it or fall down. I went to bed early and completely exhausted, thinking so much about my technique. I dreamed about snowboarding and, finally, on day three, I caught myself smiling, feeling all excited about going up in the gondola. It was a great sensation.

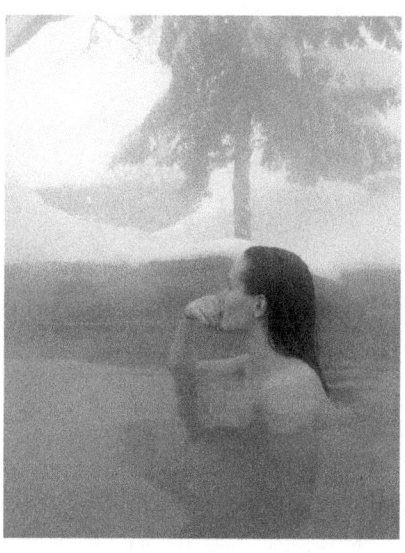

Japanese hot spring (*onsen*)

The Fear Bucket List

After a long day on the mountain, we would go and bathe in the local *onsen*, a Japanese hot spring. I remember lying on the smooth warm rocks looking up at the sky when big snowflakes started falling down. The contrast of the white snow and the hot spring was such a wonderful feeling.

Once again, I had conquered my fear and turned it into something really pleasurable. Snowboarding has become something I really look forward to.

During the rest of the week, I kept pushing myself further and further every time I started feeling sure of myself. I went faster, tried new routes, deeper powder, snowboarded in between trees, and ended up jumping a little bit. Each day I felt stronger and stronger, more in balance, and more in touch with who I really am—a conscious being, a spirit in symbiosis with nature. It was wonderful what nature and fresh air could do for you!

Chapter 17:
Fear of Public Speaking

"Do one thing every day that scares you."

Eleanor Roosevelt

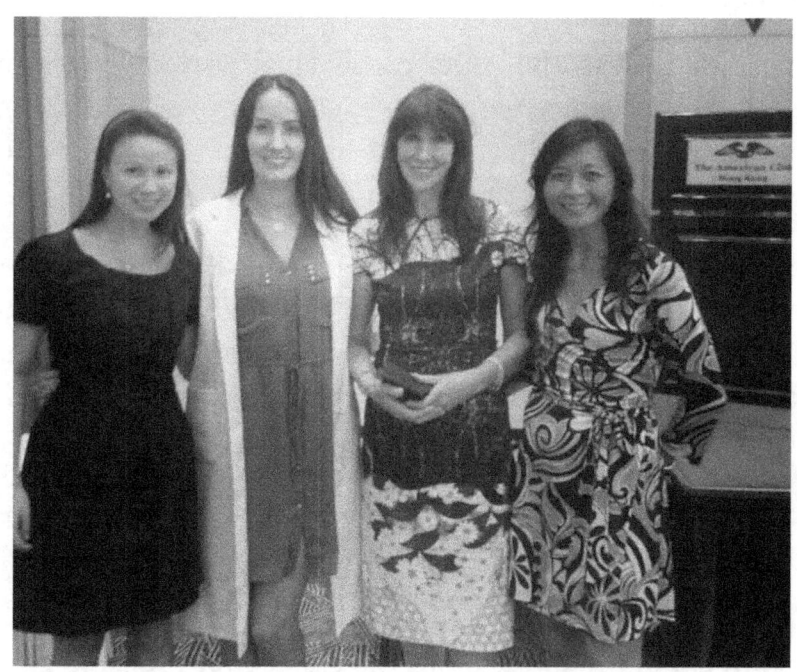

Empowering young women with
Melissa, Phyllis, and Yan-Yan

The Fear Bucket List

I was really flattered when I was invited to speak in the prestigious American Club in Hong Kong.

The point of the speaking event was to empower young women, aged eleven to fourteen, and tell them about my life and career path.

I have always been very passionate about helping others, which is why I studied chiropractic and life coaching. But, up until this day, I had only helped people one on one in the clinic.

The thought of speaking in public had always scared me, and I always avoided any kind of presentation in school growing up.

When I arrived at the American Club, I was introduced to the three other ladies who were speaking as well. They were all quite experienced, and they had prepared PowerPoint presentations and great speeches.

While I was waiting for my turn, it crossed my mind how ironic it was that I was so scared of the stage, when my sister is a Danish singer, and my extended family runs a circus. You would think I was born to perform, but no.

I was the third to speak, and I was listening to the amazing accomplishments and charity organizations the other women were involved in, when I suddenly felt my mouth go dry ... just when the microphone was handed over to me!

I had to stand up and walk to the stage, and I felt my knees trembling. I had absolutely no control over this, and I had to start my speech.

Chapter 17: Fear of Public Speaking

After a couple of seconds, I reminded myself I was there to help and just give the girls some motivation and advice, and I instantly felt less nervous and started to relax a little bit more. I found that it helped walking around a little on stage instead of standing still and really take my time to speak the words clearly. I kept saying to myself, "For Pete's sake, you have dived with white sharks; you can do this!"

The speech went well, I imagine. I don't remember much of my time on stage, but I do remember getting the girls to laugh a little, so my mission was accomplished!

I felt uplifted afterwards and humbled at the same time. I had faced my fear of public speaking and possibly motivated some young girls to make good choices in life. The best thing was that it didn't kill me.

It's a great way to get your message out there! I made it my mission to get booked on my next event within a month, in order to keep doing public speaking and challenging myself. I'm regularly being asked to come speak at events now. Who would have thought that would happen to this former introverted woman?

I still get nervous before a speaking event, but just because I'm not in my element doesn't mean I won't do it. If there is the slightest chance I can help just one woman out there, it's worth the anxiety of being on stage.

Bonus:
Advice from a Danish Singer

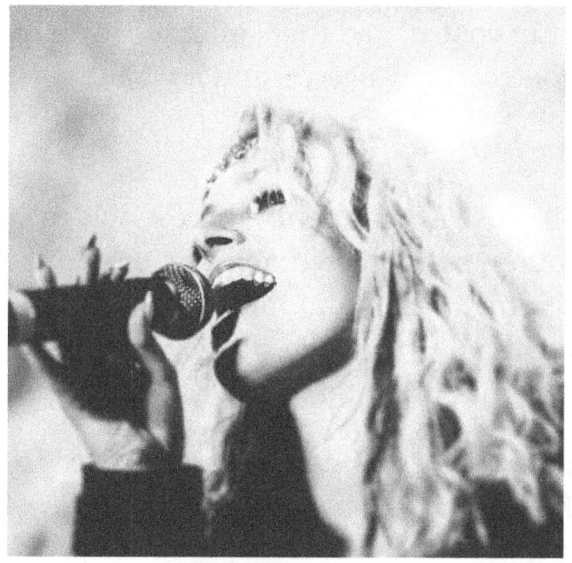

Kat Stephie

This is an interview with talented Danish singer Kat Stephie, who has many years of experience performing on stage and happens to be my baby sister. She has been on Idols and was part of the Danish pop trio Sukkerchok.

The Fear Bucket List

"How did you feel the first time you went on stage? What went through your mind? Were you scared?"

Kat: "I was scared! Of course, that has changed since, but I used to be really scared. I used to start sweating and get a feeling of being choked. I would get really hot and, sometimes, when it was really bad, I would shake a little bit too and that is very difficult when you sing, because you need the control. When your voice and body are shaking, it's very hard to control your voice. That was very bad for me in the beginning, and I always started the first couple of minutes not in control and then, after a couple of minutes, I would get control of my nerves, and it would be better."

"That sounds difficult!"

Kat: "Yes it was. I don't think there's one recipe for that type of emotion, being scared and anxious. You really have to dig deep into yourself and find the control on your own. There's no manual next to the stage saying *just breathe ten times and you'll be okay*. So, yes, it can be very difficult!"

"What do you do to prepare yourself before you go on stage? Do you have a special ritual or anything like that?"

Kat: "There are different ways to prepare. You can warm up your voice—that's the physical way to prepare—but there is also the emotional way. For me, I figured out that the more familiar I am with the material and the stuff I perform with, and the better I know the lyrics, the better I am and the less nervous I get. That is my safety net. If I have all my stuff together, it's hard to lose control. It helps me psychologically.

"Physically, I warm up, but sometimes I still forget to do this if someone asks me to sing a song at a party, and I don't have twenty minutes to go and warm up. Sometimes, when that happens, I don't have the same control over my voice. Warming up the voice is like the homework of a performer."

"How do you cope with your nerves?"

Kat: "I still get nervous when, for example, I have to impress someone in the audience. But I have discovered that if I put some of the nerves on the side, I actually don't think about it. I kind of leave my head behind the stage, because if I think too much while I'm on stage, I'm going to screw it up for myself. For me it helps to disconnect my brain emotionally. If I don't, it will really get the better of me."

"Do you have a mantra or anything else you tell yourself?"

Kat: "When I did the Danish version of the Eurovision Song Contest, I did. Right before I went on stage, I prayed for myself and the other girls who were singing, and I asked God to take my nerves away so I could have a great night. Actually, that was the biggest audience I've ever performed in front of. There were about two thousand people in the audience and about two million people watching from home on TV. It was so much fun!"

The Fear Bucket List

"How did you feel afterwards?"

Kat: "I felt amazing, because I let myself be part of the moment instead of being frozen by fear. Normally, when you do let the emotion take the best of you, you forget about the situation. But, because I stayed in the moment, I had a good recollection of what happened, and I got to relive it in a positive way."

"Do you have any other fears?"

Kat: "Yes ... I have a fear of heights; I don't like walking to the edge and looking down. There's this sushi restaurant in the Tivoli Hotel in Copenhagen on the top floor. The floor is made of glass, and I can't make myself walk over the glass, because you can see all the way down to the sidewalk."

"Do you have any fear you have overcome and gone through, even though you were scared, and how did you do it?"

Kat: "I have definitely overcome my fear of going on stage, because now I'm on stage all the time. I overcame this fear back when I was sixteen years old. I was doing a TV show called IDOLS. I was on stage so many times, I just got used to it. I remember being nervous, because I was thinking there were so many people I could disappoint if I didn't do well. So, because I had the pressure from other people and the camera in my face, I just had to do it! It wasn't because it was easy, I just got used to it after a while. If I hadn't overcome it back then, I wouldn't be where I am today!

"Other fears ... I hate spiders ... it's weird, because I love reptiles, snakes etc., but I just don't like spiders. I live a little

Bonus: Advice from a Danish Singer

house outside of the city, so the spiders are quite huge. So, if I see a spider on the ceiling, I call my husband and ask him to get rid of it. It's not that I couldn't get rid of it myself, I just don't want to kill it if it's too big. I feel like I'm taking a soul. Normally, I would run out of the room and not go back there until it was gone."

"So you acknowledge the spider is there, but you don't freak out anymore. You think about it and find a solution."

Kat: "Exactly! I'm calm and collected about it. But I still dislike the spiders."

"What advice would you give to anyone who has a fear of public speaking or performing on stage?"

Kat: "Well the first instinct you have is NOT to do it, because you don't want to put yourself in that situation. You're sweating, your palms are moist, and your heart is beating. The best advice I could ever give is to do it in spite of all that!

"You don't have to start with a big audience. You can just do it for friends and family. Normally, people who know you can be the toughest audience. They will judge you harder. Do it in front of someone you trust, so they can give you constructive feedback. And then do it many times in a row, because you will discover that every time you do it again, you will also remember some of it and free up your mind to think of different stuff.

"I don't believe in the old myth of imagining the audience naked. I think that is so weird, and it would make me even

The Fear Bucket List

more nervous to think about undressing people in the room! But I do believe *the more you do it, the better it will get*. And I would say *be calm*, even though you'll be nervous the first time you do it in front of a lot of people.

"*Accept it* and just sit down after you're done and write down what was good, what was bad, and *analyze it*, so you can make it better the next time. Even though you have ten bad things on your list and only five good things, and even though you can only make just one of the ten bad things better, it's still a win situation for you, because you have taken a small step in the right direction.

"There are so many talented people out there, with so many great things on their mind, but they don't say it, because they have this fear of speaking. So, think about how many people you can help by speaking and just do it! *Don't think too much; just do it!*"

Conclusion

"The journey of facing your fears is like cave diving in halocline layers. At first it's clear, but then it gets foggy and your visibility disappears, sometimes only for a moment, but sometimes for several meters. If you stop, you'll stay in the dark but, if you continue on your path, you'll reach the light at the end."

Dr. Kamilla Holst

This Is Not the End.
It Is the Beginning!

Facing your fears is an ongoing process. I'm still working on my Fear Bucket List, but each thing I cross off that list brings me closer to my spirit and, as a result, a higher consciousness and inner peace.

It empowers me as a human being and gives me tools to teach others. It gives me experiences for life and adventures to look forward to. It reminds me, that life is a journey, and I choose the meaning of it all.

Facing your fears is a great method of connecting to your inner self. The more you do this, the stronger you become!

My point is **if I can do this, you can too**! Whether it's skydiving, public speaking, or swimming with sharks, you need the self-discipline to do something you don't really like or want to do, and do it anyway!

The *hidden benefits* (that I didn't expect at all) of facing the fears on my Fear Bucket List were an inner peace, a sense of love, and a presence that everyone around me notices. My relationship is better. I feel safe and loved. The guilt and self-doubt has disappeared. It transformed me into a power woman!

The hardest part for me on this journey was not the action-packed things on my Fear Bucket List. Those experiences really helped me take back my power and elevate my consciousness. Learning how to trust a man again, open my heart to the masculine energy, and trust that not all men are bad was the hardest part, and I'm still working on that every day with my man.

He is the kindest, most generous, and patient man I have ever met, and he helps me heal all my traumas by being there for me. He respects me and doesn't feel the need to dominate me to feel superior. He has taught me how to receive love and pleasure without pain—something I never thought would be possible. He talks to me and tries to understand how I'm feeling inside when I have my bad days, which still happens from time to time.

Venturing outside of your comfort zone and taking positive risks is a great way to help you feel more positive about yourself, encourage a positive change in your life, and build your confidence.

Sometimes you will fail, it is inevitable, but, hey, many successful people make mistakes and start over several times before they reach their potential.

Even when it feels like everything is taken away from you and you have to start all over again, this is a gift. It empowers you. It makes you who you are.

This Is Not the End. It Is the Beginning!

Now is the time to face your fears more than ever and pull yourself up one step at a time. Doing scary things is a great way to empower yourself on this journey, as well as learning to look inwards and establish that inner connection again with the help from meditation.

All in all, human emotions can be broken down into *love* and *fear*.

Love heals everything and love is all there is. That is the lesson we are supposed to learn.

It might take several lifetimes, or you can make a short cut by eliminating your fear and other feelings that eventually lead to fear.

Fear is the absence of love. Fear attracts whatever it is you fear. Really remember this, where your focus goes, your energy flows, so stop yourself from worrying all the time. Be aware of the undercurrent of thoughts you have on a daily basis and try to replace the negative ones with positive healing thoughts instead. You can teach your brain to do this by starting a gratitude journal, writing down every day all the things you are grateful for in your life. That way you teach your brain to find the positive instead of the negative.

Remember, fear is temporary ... and it carries with it opportunities to learn, to grow, and to expand. Look at the lessons and opportunities in it and focus on what you want!

Our true self is fearless!

Know that worrying is just another way of fear, and it creates negative images in our mind and creates doubt. It's an unnecessary spiral, yet many of us still spend a lot of time worrying.

My advice is to learn to cherish the unknown. Get out of your comfort zone! Let go of your need to control. This is where the joy and happiness lies. Trust your spirit.

"Acknowledging your fear is key. It will not just go away by itself; you have to learn how to deal with it when it occurs."

Frogman Georg H. Petersen 'Putte'

I have given you some examples in my book of how to face your fears, and it really doesn't matter what kind of fear you have, the principle is the same. Just <u>face your fear</u>, <u>don't think too much</u>, and <u>jump right into it</u> like a child. The next time it won't be so scary. Don't let the fear take over your life and keep you trapped. You deserve better than that!

Sometimes, all we need is to make a decision, follow through with it, and not let anything deter us.

We all face different challenges, but remember, no matter what has happened to you in the past, **it is always up to you to decide how you're going to live your life.** Are you going to live in fear, be a victim, blame others, and stay stuck, or are you going to take responsibility for your life, believe in yourself, and choose the path of awakening and freedom?

Instead of beating yourself up and feeling guilty about the past, think "I was acting on the best information I had at the time, given the state I was in." Learn to forgive and let go.

This Is Not the End. It Is the Beginning!

You can use this mantra:

"I believe that I attract exactly what I need in order for my spirit to develop and learn what it is I'm here to learn. I accept everything that comes my way, no matter how scary it might seem in the moment, because I know there are just as many great experiences and happy events on my journey as well, if I dare to overcome my fears and move forward."

By having the courage to identify and confront your fears, you grant yourself the power to transcend, creating freedom, happiness, and absolute bliss. All fear can be eliminated, given time.

Eventually the fear will pass, the fear every human being carries with them in this life, and you will feel free to live your life on your own terms. You will feel really alive and naturally elevate your own consciousness to a higher level, just like the initiates did in ancient Egypt.

The best way to get over fear, is to face it and embrace it!

The only limitations we have are the ones we put on ourselves. Life is created for our enjoyment, self-discovery, and learning, so don't let fear stop you.

***

Now, it's your turn, <u>I challenge you</u>, to create your own journey of awakening and write down your own Fear Bucket List!

"The only thing to fear is fear itself!"

Winston Churchill

I would love to connect with you and hear your story, please join my Facebook Group - share your Fear Bucket List and what fears you have already overcome or are planning to overcome:

www.facebook.com/TheFearBucketList

DrHolst@TheFearBucketList.com

And if you know someone who could benefit from the information in this book, please pass it along to them!

Go to www.TheFearBucketList.com to download your workbook.

This Is Not the End. It Is the Beginning!

Exercise:

List below what you would be able to accomplish if you were fearless.

-

-

-

What would your life be like?

MY FEAR BUCKET LIST

1.

2.

3.

4.

5.

6.

7.

8.

9.

10.

Exercise:

Ask yourself these questions and write your answers down:

Where are you in your life right now?

Is something holding you back?

Do you have a secret?

What can you do today to change your life?

Be honest with yourself and write down your top three fears here:

1.

2.

3.

References

Chaudhary, Sufian. *World of Archangels*. 2013

Chopra, Deepak. *Perfect Health*. 1990

Covey, Stephen. *The 7 Habits of Highly Effective People*. 1989

Germain, Maureen J. St. *Beyond The Flower of Life*. 2009

Gray, Henry. *Gray's Anatomy*. 1858.

Hay, Louise. *Heal Your Body*. 1976

Madanes, Cloé. *Relationship Breakthrough: How to Create Outstanding Relationships in Every Area of Your Life*. 2009

Madanes, Cloé. *Sex, Love and Violence: Strategies for Transformation*. 1990.

Madsen, Anders Lund. *Dr. Zukarovs Testamente*. 2012

Manzini, Fabrizio. *The Power of Self-healing*. 2012

Melchiezedek, Drunvalo. *The Ancient Secret of the Flower of Life*. 1999.

Netter, Frank H. *Atlas of Human Anatomy*. 1989

O'connor and Seymour. *Introducing Neuro-linguistic Programming*. 2002.

Robbins, Anthony. *Awaken the Giant Within*. 2007

Robbins, Anthony. *Unlimited Power*. 2008

Schmidt, Daniel. Documentary: *Inner Worlds, Outer Worlds – Part 4 – Beyond Thinking*. 2012

Tolle, Eckhart. *The Power of Now*. 2004

Wilde, Stuart. *Life Was Never Meant To Be a Struggle*. 1987

Wilde, Stuart. *Infinite Self*. 1996

www.arkofhopeforchildren.org

www.google.com

www.hagarinternational.org

www.rainn.org

www.wikipedia.org

Zukav, Gary. *The Seat of the Soul*. 1989

Zukav, Gary. *Spiritual Partnership*. 2000

Acknowledgments

Thank you to my spiritual guides and the archangels for helping me write this book.

I'm very grateful for the kind endorsements from around the world. A special thanks to Cloé Madanes, Sofia Manning, Melissa Petros, and Sufian Chaudhary.

Thanks to Maureen Saint Germain for inspiring me and guiding me when I needed to finish my book by opening up my Akashic records and thank you for your endorsement.

Thank you Reiki master Margit Moelgaard for your friendship and mentorship, not to mention our many tea sessions in Denmark.

Thank you to my teachers from Ladakh; Buddhist monk Chokyong Palga Tulku Rinpoche, from Hong Kong; tai chi master Dr. Benjamin Yip; and, from Mexico, Mayan elder Don Pedro Pablo Chuc.

Thanks to my man for allowing me to believe in love again, supporting me, and taking care of me when I needed it the most.

Thanks to my mother and sister for their continuous support and guidance, keeping it real, and being true to themselves always—my power women!

A special thanks to my frogman father for sharing his near-death experiences and life wisdom with me.

The Fear Bucket List

Thank you to my closest Hong Kong friends Ainslie, Ana R, Amanda, Joanna & Willo for being a constant inspiration to me and giving me feedback on my book in the early stages.

And last, but not least, thank you for your trust to all the patients I have had the pleasure of healing already and my loyal tribe on social media—you are my purpose. Let's change the world together one soul at a time.

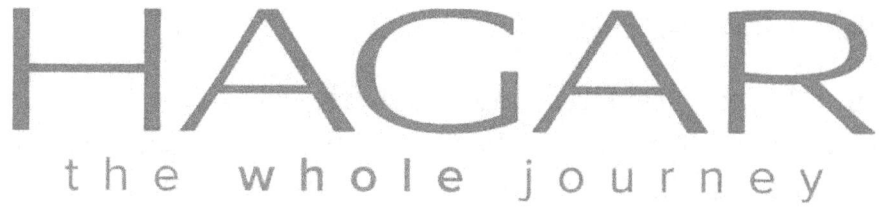

About Hagar International

www.hagarinternational.org

Hagar International is a non-profit organization that specializes in restoring and empowering women and children in Afghanistan, Cambodia, and Vietnam whose lives have been devastated by extreme human rights abuses—particularly domestic violence, exploitation, and human trafficking. Since 1994, Hagar has helped over 20,000 survivors.

Hagar uses a holistic, long-term approach that addresses the unique and complex needs of each survivor that enters our care. Hagar's programs are conducted through the lens of our five domains of change, which we believe are essential in fostering life-changing transformations for survivors.

<u>Protection</u>

Hagar works to ensure each survivor's safety in our shelters, centers, and community-based care options in the countries we work. Additionally, our Legal and Protection Unit provides legal support to survivors called to testify in court including educating them on their rights and how to protect themselves.

Personal Well-Being

In Hagar's centers and shelters, survivors receive healthcare, trauma counseling, and nurturing, which develops their internal strength and resilience. As a result, survivors cultivate the ability to "bounce back" or even grow in the face of adversity, trauma, or tragedy.

Economic Empowerment

Through catch-up schooling, life skills education, career counseling, vocational training, and job placements, Hagar helps survivors increase their power over economic decisions that influence their lives and enable greater freedom of action. Survivors are then able to start a secure and productive life where they are financially independent.

Social Capital

Hagar supports survivors as they integrate back into a community of their choice. Through a range of options including family care, community foster families, and group homes, Hagar helps each survivor build healthy relationships with their family, friends, and community.

Societal Change

Hagar advocates, educates, and conducts innovative research to help governments, civil society, and communities strengthen protection frameworks for survivors. Through these partnerships, Hagar influences positive systemic and societal change with and on behalf of survivors on the journey towards protection and recovery.

About Dr. Kamilla Holst

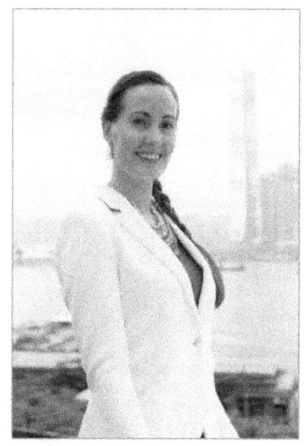 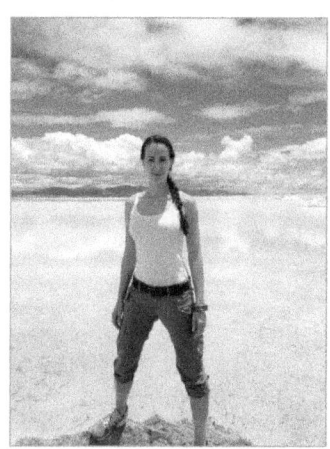

Dr. Kamilla Holst is a qualified chiropractor and certified life coach who specializes in providing a holistic treatment to women.

In 2014, Dr. Holst relocated from Denmark to Hong Kong where she is considered the go-to pregnancy chiropractor.

Throughout her career, she has treated thousands of people, and she continues to teach her patients the importance of self-healing and body/mind balance.

Find out more about Kamilla's work on her websites and join her Facebook group and Instagram communities.

DrHolst@TheFearBucketList.com

www.TheFearBucketList.com

www.kamillaholst.com

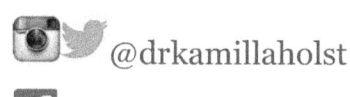 @drkamillaholst

/TheFearBucketList

www.ingramcontent.com/pod-product-compliance
Lightning Source LLC
Chambersburg PA
CBHW061437180526
45170CB00004B/1450